Treating Autism with Bumetanide

Treating Autism with Bumetanide

By

Yehezkel Ben-Ari, Eric Lemonnier and Nouchine Hadjikhani

Cambridge Scholars Publishing

Treating Autism with Bumetanide

By Yehezkel Ben-Ari, Eric Lemonnier and Nouchine Hadjikhani

This book first published 2023

Cambridge Scholars Publishing

Lady Stephenson Library, Newcastle upon Tyne, NE6 2PA, UK

British Library Cataloguing in Publication Data
A catalogue record for this book is available from the British Library

ISBN (10): 1-5275-1890-6
ISBN (13): 978-1-5275-1890-2

https://leblogdebenari.com/

CONTENTS

FOREWORD

Discoveries are the product of a complex recipe requiring experience, hard work, patience, highly instructive errors that must not be ignored and the capacity of going beyond established dogmas to create novel concepts that in due time will be challenged by next generation. Knowledge evolves by unpredictable steps with most of us contributing small increments and one of our successors having the intuition and the talent to draw from our observations far reaching conclusions that we failed to consider. There is, however, also a chance factor, meetings with colleagues and changing environment impacts our vision and facilitates the emergence of intuition – an ill-defined term that is relevant to step forward advances. When Fleming discovered penicillin, he did not look askance at the bacteria that failed to grow next to a particular fungus. Rather, he was ripe for observing the unexpected, which might lead him down new avenues of research and treatment. Passion rewards the original researchers who study their surroundings with a fresh gaze. Intuition, a quality fashioned from knowledge, experience, and a generous helping of curiosity, can lead the lucky to the top of creativity. At the end of the day, chance smiles to those who are aware and ripe to harvest the fruits!

The icing on the cake is that these discoveries often lead to a questioning of established concepts. For a scientist, that is the Holy Grail. Science is never set in stone, anything at any time can be questioned, and this everlasting process is its fuel for growth. Science does not do well under rigidity and strict programming. Numerous examples illustrate how guided, and sterile research has a low probability of fostering qualitative leaps in knowledge. All the tools that are now part of our daily life – from the theory of relativity and its applications a century later, to X-ray, imaging, discoveries in genetics, stem cells, transplants, antidepressants, GPS, e-mail, radar – are the product of minds that were ahead of their time, of theories that were considered zany before becoming obvious. Along the way, some of those responsible for new discoveries ended up incarcerated. Defeat is orphaned whilst success has many parents. The road is littered with pitfalls. There is the conservatism of those who oppose all questioning. The temple keepers are scientific research's perennial nemesis. Then, there are financial interests, which influence the direction of science depending on the importance attached to the field by the global economy at any given time. Contrary to common belief, science is not neutral, ethereal nor flavourless; it is the product of women and men who are prey to their egos, to fashions, to power relations, and to dominant forces. Science is becoming exceedingly expensive, increasing researchers' dependency on those who hold the purse strings. This state of affairs is at the root of numerous false discoveries, the lifespan of which is but the length of a sigh. Their discoverers are bestowed with a moment of media exposure, fame, and ephemeral honour. It is the era of Kleenex researchers, like the pop singers who beguile teenagers for a handful of weeks. Yet passion remains indispensable as a fuel of discovery.

This story is the product of an encounter between a biophysics researcher passionate about understanding the mechanisms governing brain maturation and a psychiatrist who seeks to treat autism, one of the most debilitating developmental disorders. The researcher tries to understand the role genes and the environment play in brain formation (the innate and the conditioned) and how neural pathways develop. He does not have a diagnostic or therapeutic goal in mind. Rather, he is guided by curiosity, which acts as both compass and talisman. The psychiatrist wants to enter the bubble within which afflicted children enclose themselves. In the face of this trying disorder, parents often latch onto false hopes. He is guided by permanent suffering, life stories, and the despair of parents who have no handbook to help them understand their inability to communicate with their children. In short, the breadth and boundaries of neuropsychiatry.

This unexpected meeting will create a dialogue between two parallel worlds that usually ignore each other. Researchers are seen as spoiled children who allow themselves the luxury of virtual reality and abstract questions, whereas psychiatrists bring support *hic et nunc*. The present is brought face to face with the promises of a possible future – definitely a difficult dialogue to foster. A common language develops around a passion for understanding and treatment. A presumably crazy idea is born from this meeting: to treat autism with a diuretic. A third person then joins the two, someone just as iconoclastic, an expert in brain imaging persuaded that visualising brain activity can help us identify the afflicted neural networks and their footprint. An ideal approach that allows us to move from animals to humans better than any other method, a bit like a painter who continuously retouches the same canvas.

Indirect and potentially simplistic observations have helped the basic science expert to detect high concentrations of chloride in the nerve cells of immature neurons but also in adult neurons recorded in animal models of a large number of brain disorders including epilepsies, brain trauma, spinal cord injuries, infract and chronic pain. These observations suggest that insults produce neurons endowed somehow with immature features – a sort of return to the future! A complex situation endowed with numerous philosophical, experimental and even ethical issues. It is, however also endowed with possible novel common therapies to treat for many neurological and psychiatric disorders. This is counterintuitive as these disorders have different aetiologies, clinical manifestations and outcome. Yet, if high levels of neuronal chloride are observed in these disorders, then a diuretic known to reduce neuronal chloride might be used to attenuate them. As we cannot determine chloride levels in neurons in children with autism (this is best performed in vitro in brain slices!), it is instrumental to rely on experimental animals that mimic autism either by administration of a drug or a genetic mutation associated with autism in humans. Usually, basic science that requires years to provide a possible treatment precedes clinical trials. However, the reformulation of a widely-used molecule to treat another disorder that the initial one considerably shortens this latency. Diuretics have been used for decades to treat hypertension and oedemas, by reducing chloride concentrations in the kidneys and their side effects have been extensively documented simplifying the quest for approval from health authorities to perform trials. Consequently, we faced a very unusual situation where the trials were performed well before experimental data in animal models confirmed that neurons have high chloride levels and the diuretic attenuates the clinical and electrographic signatures of the disease. However, the combination of clinical and experimental observations is instrumental as the improvement of a clinical symptom in children by a drug does not imply that the suspected mechanism is the correct one! There are several alternative possibilities that must be taken into consideration (see below).

The idea to treat autism with a simple molecule with diuretic properties annoys geneticists, who are convinced that autism is genetic and that it will only be diagnosed and treated once the hundreds of mutations sometimes associated with it are identified. It does not matter to them that the 'gene' for autism cannot be found, nor that the hundreds of mutations concern only a small percentage of those with the disorder, nor that to identify the mutation would not bring us any closer to treating it. 'We will make it' they sing in unison and in blind faith. Our era desires this, the certainty that everything, or nearly everything, is genetically determined: intelligence, foolishness, personality, behaviour, religious belief, sexuality, aggression or criminality. Of course, neurological and psychiatric disorders fall under this spell, a chain of genetic and epigenetic events that lose their mystery, bringing forth healing and improvement. And tomorrow, pigs will fly!

Historically, not very long time ago, the other extreme was filled by the ayatollahs of psychoanalytic sophistry – and this to some extent is still very much the case in France and French speaking countries. Largely disconnected from biological reality and floating in the ether, it seems that the only justification for their approach is to ensure that their caste becomes perennial – to the detriment of the patients. Here, biology, randomised clinical trials and statistics are barbaric terms reserved for use by narrow-minded scientists. But the evidence speaks for itself and only ignorant people will claim that autism is a disorder reflecting a mother's supposed lack of desire for a child. We will, therefore, scrutinise the distant past with a telescope in search of the trigger. Bettelheim has popped by, mixing concentration camps, phallus, the desire to procreate, maternal love, grandiose language and academic discourse. When we try to remind these clinicians that there is a biology of molecules behind all this, a malformation of the brain, and children who do not even master language when the disorder is in its first stages, they still reply that speaking heals and that *we* are the ignorant ones who have forgotten the separation between mind and body. They insist on viewing these molecules and biochemical processes without cure with snobbery. The source is again and always childhood, troubled relationships with the mother, sexuality – the general hullabaloo of psychoanalysis. Speaking is sufficient in itself; it does not require experimental proof. The majesty of speech and beautiful phrasing: French sickness *par excellence*. Descartes is obviously the export product; a prophet hath no honour in his own country. Admittedly, this is now less accepted because science has progressed, yet, at times when fake news become prevalent, other vicious attacks of scientific observations challenging the usefulness of vaccines suggested to cause autism have emerged. This is indeed an endless fight! Elsewhere, pragmatism dominates and, like Saint Thomas we only believe what we see and luckily psychoanalysis became out of fashion in most countries at least as far as autism in children is concerned.

Admittedly, the genetic reductionism that exaggerates the therapeutic benefits it brings has played a decisive role in this abandon and helped the mother to get rid of the guilt that dominated a couple of decades ago. Yet, the discovery of mutations compellingly associated with "simple" monogenic disorders – like Huntington's disease or the Duchesne dystrophy – has not led to suitable treatments! The principal reason for this failure is that, as will be discussed below, the plasticity of brain networks responds to insults by modifications that disrupt the simplistic link between one gene and the disease. The superficial link one gene – one protein – one disorder ignores the essential roles of development, life conditions and environmental factors that translate the gene to a given outcome in most cases. Homeric struggle leaves little room for a third voice: those who want neither option. The two sides rally against those who seek to understand how neural networks function in the face of adversity. After all, if there has been a communication breakdown, we should expect traces of it in neural networks' electric activity that generates the brain's rhythms.

Is that debate truly devoid of an ideological approach? The situation is further complicated by the fact that autism is not like other disorders. First, it seems to be affecting an increasing number of people – more than 1% in the last epidemiological studies. Second, it combines elements that are particularly sensitive to us: a handicap that originates in the womb and the first few years of childhood, affecting communication and socialising, aspects at the heart of modern society. Since early diagnosis is difficult and cures do not exist, the inability to communicate at an early age creates a vicious cycle that invalidates this crucial stage in life when we adapt to society. Moreover, because autism has a wide range of symptoms, it is difficult to understand its mechanisms and to develop new therapies. Autism has been linked to a plethora of factors, from the mother's or father's age to birth issues (preterm delivery, programmed caesarean, delivery complications, anoxic periods…), and a lot of environmental factors. In brief, a disorder with an early start, a history characterised by variable geometry, cumulating genetic and environmental factors… A nightmare situation for the researcher and the clinician but a boon for swindlers.

Our story will present why a diuretic, which has been prescribed for four decades to treat hypertension and cerebral oedema, can be used to improve the quality of the life of children (and adults) with autism and that of their parents by extension. This conclusion has its roots in a theoretical concept and experimental data. It has been fostered by the wonderful decision of a brain imaging expert to join the team and her demonstration that treatment normalized crucial areas of the brain linked to social and emotional processing. Thus, we escape murky water, whilst in parallel, less constraining data has shown us that high chloride concentrations exist in the model neurons of autistic animals. From there, the fight involves overcoming administrative difficulties and finding the right financing to create a treatment adapted to autistic children. This story highlights the difficult practices of the biomedical world, which are characterised by the medical and scientific fields' conservatism, and the axiomatic slowness and grotesque bureaucracy that must be conquered to successfully develop a drug.

It is not an exaggeration to state that our efforts to develop a novel treatment based on a diuretic – in spite of the compelling experimental observations and clinical trials, have been met with profound skepticism. Many psychiatrists considered this almost as fake news, papers published on the difficulty to develop novel medicaments and their inefficacy did not even mention our successful trials. From the basic science world, things have been slightly but not significantly better. Somehow, conservatism to novel ideas prevails. To convince, we needed far more basic and clinical data than was required from other approaches more in accord with the dominating modes – we will show that this is what we did.

It goes without saying that our main reason for writing is the parents' experience. It is to them that we dedicate this book. They are the true heroes, who retain trust in science and progress and fuel our passion to overcome all obstacles. Moving on from these testimonies, we attempt to convince the reader that a healthy measure of humility is necessary when we are dealing with such a complex illness. There cannot be a solution as simple as the aspirin used to cure a headache. This is because autism's early origins mean its symptoms cannot be completely erased. But parents are themselves describing the treatment's benefits: 'Our child is more present.' Our book will devote its better part to the testimonies of autistic children and their families.

To contextualise the problem, we will first summarise the mechanisms that govern the brain and its construction and how they can go wrong, giving rise to neurological and psychiatric disorders. Then, we will present the main points on autism, before moving on to the findings from our therapeutic trials and the critical input from brain imaging. The testimonies from autistic children and their parents will allow us to explore the treatment's benefits and its limits.

I

THE EXTRAORDINARY STORY OF THE BRAIN'S CONSTRUCTION

1. Neurons, synapses, neural networks, and ionic currents

The brain. It is a complex organ, which receives, analyses, and integrates information, memorising some of it and producing a response that takes into account both recent and not-so-recent history. This occurs through the intermediary of neurons and the synapses that interconnect them, creating functional networks composed of millions and sometimes billions of neurons working in concert to generate brain activity. This activity will translate into the responses we have to our environment: our behaviour.

Neurons. These are cells specialised in the reception of information and its transformation first into chemical signals and then into electrical ones. Their activity is propagated via hundreds of millions of synaptic connections and will be translated into behaviour, reaction, and memory… A neuron is a cell with positive and negative ion charges, a bit like a battery that generates electrical current via negative and positive electrolytes. An essential part of its energy is used to preserve ionic gradients between its interior and the exterior.

Neurons have elongations, dendrites, and axon. Myriad types of neurons exist. They are always made up of a core, the cell body, and tree-like elongations. The dendrites and the axon extend from the cell body, constituting respectively the start and end of the neuron. The electrical activity reaches the dendrites and then propagates towards the cell body and the axon to transmit the information to the neuron's target. Information is analysed at every step of the transmission.

The synapses. These are points of contact and of information transmission between two nerve cells. They are also the main location for the integration of our activities, their analysis, memory building, and all the properties that allow our brain to be such a high-performing and flexible machine. They are the true heart of our integrative capacity. Defective synapses are a sign of numerous brain disorders, autism included. The human brain is made up of thousands of billions of synapses. Comparing the brain's complexity to the processing power of a mobile phone puts this in perceptive. To achieve the brain's complexity, each person would have to carry hundreds of thousands of mobile phones. We understand the organisational difficulty and functioning of this hub, but how does it actually work?

Synaptic transmission. The arrival of an electrical influx into the terminals of a nerve cell will unleash a chemical mediator that will be recognised by the target cell and will generate an ionic current. This current will, in turn, act on the targets of this neuron. The activation of a synapse and the transfer of information to its target lasts a few thousandths of a second, a delay that incorporates the release of the mediator, the activation of target structures and the genesis by the target cell of an electric current that will propagate towards other targets. Synapses are the true heart of our brain's functioning. It is therefore important to understand its functioning and its anomalies. To regulate brain activity and to generate discharge patterns in addition to the associated behaviours, neurons have excitatory and inhibitory synapses that act a bit like a brake and an accelerator. On the one hand, the brain must maintain a constant equilibrium between brake and accelerator and, on the other, it must produce rhythms at specific times that correspond to particular brain activities.

Chemical mediators. We are aware of a number of chemical mediators but two principal ones govern most of the field: glutamate and GABA. They are both synthesised in distinct neural groupings and exercise complementary roles in the behaviour-generation factory. The glutamatergic neurons, which release glutamate, are the most common. The release of glutamate into the synaptic space is recognised by the target neuron's receptors and triggers excitatory currents of positively charged ions called cations. The introduction of cations (sodium, potassium or calcium) will decrease the target cell's rest potential and will excite it. The GABAergic neurons that release GABA are less common (representing between 10% and 20% of neurons). The release of GABA translates into inhibitory currents in the target cell, which are generated by negatively charged ions called anions, of which chloride is a well-known example. The introduction of chloride into the target cell will increase the rest potential – charging the battery, if you will – and the cell will have trouble generating an excitatory response. These synapses are therefore inhibitory because they tend to reduce the target cells' activity. The GABA synapses are the target of many tranquilising and treatment molecules, such as benzodiazepines (Valium®), barbiturates and other anaesthetics and anxiolytics. They work by increasing the efficiency of GABAergic currents and reducing brain activity enough to produce their calming effects. We therefore understand how neurons must constantly control the equilibrium between excitation and inhibition, knowing that if excitation dominates or if inhibition is depleted, the network will overexcite and, for example, generate epileptic fits.

Brain oscillations. These are electrical activities generated by groups of neurons connected by synapses. The oscillations reflect at once the networks' analyses, the integration of information included in these analyses, and the expression of the corresponding behaviours. Adult brains constantly generate oscillations usually defined by their frequency (cycles per seconds, or Hertz), which range from a few cycles per second to tens of cycles per second and sometimes more, especially in pathological situations. Thus, brain oscillations signal what we do and the behaviour that results from it.

2. The main phases of brain development

The brain's complexity has increased throughout evolution. The main phases in its development are clear and consist of five principal moments.

The formation of a neural tube. During embryogenesis, a tube is formed with cells encircling it. It has dorsal and frontal poles, and dorsal and frontal faces. The general schema has remained the same since our oldest ancestors.

The proliferation. To generate the countless number of nerve cells that will make up the brain, the cells divide following a set rate and schema. A modification in the duration of cell division and/or the period during which the cells divide can change the result dramatically. We indeed think that evolution has partly developed through such variations. Nerve cells are generated in excess and the number will adjust itself during a period of time lasting until puberty. Thus, our cortex can lose many thousands of cells and millions of synapses per minute (as we will see below). Once the final number of cells has been reached, they stop regenerating themselves, save for those located in the central structures (olfactory cells and the neurons of the dentate gyrus). Contrary to the publicity surrounding this subject, which is as mistaken as it is pervasive, our cortical cells do not renew themselves, and the brain is not a fountain of eternal youth. There are genetic disorders caused by mutations that alter the proliferation, giving rise to an excess of neurons, like autism, or to fewer neurons, like certain forms of early-onset epilepsy and brain malformations.

Neural migration. Our cortex, the most developed structure in *homo sapiens*, simultaneously generates our language and our species' extraordinary integrative capacity. Although not larger than whales and other cetaceans, it has the largest surface and volume relative to our closest cousins, the chimpanzee, and is composed of six neural layers with precise organisation, composition and connections.

To build this six-storey building, we need scaffolding, an elevator, and automatic guidance control so that the elements can migrate to their assigned location. The neurons will take the lift, transforming into specialised cells called radial glial cells, and head downstairs to their assigned location. The elevator always starts by bringing the cells that reside in the lower floors and then those closer to the surface. Changes in this migration process causes severe developmental problems, such as certain mental disabilities, double cortex syndrome and tuberous sclerosis.

Differentiation. Nerve cells specialise only once they have reached their 'floor'. At which point they acquire cellular, morphological, and biochemical properties, which differentiates them into one of the thousands of cell types present in the brain.

Sprouting, the formation of synapses and neural networks. At this stage, the neurons sprout, emitting axons and dendrites (as we saw earlier) and connecting specifically with the neurons that will be part of the same functional entity. The selectivity is absolute: we can see the extensions coming into contact with a neuron, deciding that it is not the right target and moving on to find the correct one. As soon as the contact is chosen, synapses form and the two neurons will act in concert. The cellular entity is connected by millions of synapses, creating a functional whole responsible for the integration of information and/or the genesis of a particular response. At each stage, a mechanism can be defective, which can give rise to repercussions that are often severe and that can cause neurological and psychological disorders. Thus, either an excessive or insufficient proliferation will take place, which will be translated into an anarchical organisation of part of the brain that can lead to intellectual deficiency and epilepsy. A flawed migration of nerve cells can also create a double cortex. This will generate atypical activity that prevents the brain from functioning properly and give rise to severe epileptic fits that are resistant to all treatments save that of successfully removing the double cortex surgically.

To summarise, the brain's construction is organised around essential meeting points that must follow a precise timing. Any delay will lead to costly malformations, which cause many severely debilitating conditions. The genetic programme is at the heart of this construction and modulated at every step by information received from the earliest stages of its construction. The brain, when forming, is neither blind nor deaf. It is not on autopilot; it is paying attention to its environment and taking it into account as it forms its neural networks.

3. Brain maturation is controlled by genes and the environment

How is an organ as complex as the brain built? What role do genetics and the environment play in this process?

The brain's volume is between 1,200 and 1,300 m^3, three times that of our close cousins, the chimpanzees. It is the result of a true evolutionary leap in the animal kingdom. Evolution is both qualitative and quantitative. Important regions in the brain are developed preferentially. A good example is the cortical envelope and its associated cortices, which congregate information so that it can be contextualised. It took less than two million years to evolve and this evolution did not occur continuously. Instead, it developed by specialisation, as can be seen by the lack of continuity present between animal species. Thanks to this, *homo sapiens* is a social animal that can gather knowledge and use it collectively to benefit others. Humans are less sensitive to genetic determinism than their close cousins. This is because our intellect is not the result of a hyper-constrained genetic programme but is instead the consequence of complex interactions in which the environment played a crucial role.

Carrying out such a programme is not simple. For example, we need millions of ganglion cells to extend from the retina to the optical centres. This requires green and red lights and stop signs to guide the neurons' axons across the median line towards their goal. If the retinal axons do not reach their target, which happens with some genetic mutations, the visual system will not build itself. Consequently, numerous genetic mutations can make it impossible for this complex programme to develop correctly.

That being said, the genetic programme is not everything. During its construction in the uterus, the embryo listens, perceives and vibrates in response to its surroundings. The construction of its cortices is modulated by the electrical activity generated by its sensory organs, and this before any precise perception is possible. We open our eyes very early on during pregnancy, towards the end of the first trimester, and our retina is active while forming, though sight is not yet possible nor does it correspond to any visual activity. This electrical activity that is observed in a wide range of animal species from frogs to chimpanzees and humans is nevertheless important because, if we block it *in utero*, the visual centres fail to develop properly. They maintain their scheduled organisation, but this organisation lacks context and visual capacity.

How to translate and illustrate this situation? When building a car or a plane, the elements are assembled and, when all is ready, we pump in the petrol and start the engine for the first time. In contrast, the brain works from the earliest phases of its building, as if the airplane or the car already had the motor running from the first phases of construction. A very long breaking-in period follows, which will continue in part for the rest of our lifetime. Today, we know that the immature brain is very active on an electrical level, including during the early stages. Immature cells generate electrical activity that plays a crucial role in the brain's construction. *In utero* the little one is moving, exciting itself and generating an impressive amount of activity, as mothers know well. The studies we have undertaken for three decades on the brains of rodents or primates have allowed us to describe the sequences of maturation of brain activity. These activities are specific to the developing brain and are not observed in the adult one. In other words, the brain speaks a lot as it builds itself, but with a language different to that of the adult's. The data also highlights how important it is that specific drugs are developed for babies, rather than simply administering reduced doses of drugs developed for adults.

The general rule is that ionic currents are slow, which means fast signals like those needed by the adult brain for day-to-day activities (walking, driving, responding to external stimuli…) cannot be generated. It is nevertheless enough for the needs of a developing network. The developing brain is extraordinarily heterogeneous and must coordinate neurons that are at different stages of maturation so they can work together. Remember that the neurons in the human cortex are dividing during roughly a hundred days (approximately between the 40th and the 140th day of gestation). Consequently, they must cohabit and discharge together, despite some already having hundreds of synapses while others have a few or even none.

The slow currents generated by immature neurons are a perfect way of making these very different neurons work together. It is a bit like a gigantic symphony orchestra, one that is many thousands of times larger than that required playing Berlioz's *Symphonie fantastique*. During rehearsals, the members of the orchestra organise themselves by resemblance in small groups, which play pieces that are very different to the symphony. Actually, each group plays a pre-planned baroque minuet in perfect execution. When the time comes, the orchestra comes together to play the symphony without preparation. The quality of the concert will depend on the quality of the execution of the minuet by each little group. If the groups give a poor performance, the overall recital of Berlioz's symphony will be a dud. The embryo's brain harmonises these minuets, which are generated by a giant, heterodox orchestra that is seemingly without any kind of organisation, and translates it into a musical work intelligible to adult ears.

What purpose do immature minuets serve? Another analogy will help us answer this. During the construction of a building or a bridge, we proceed first by choosing an architect and a programme of works, armed with a plan and many details – this is the genetic programme. Then the work is delegated and construction site meetings ensure that it all develops as planned. The programme is checked constantly throughout the process. Thus, in the case of the Channel tunnel, building works were undertaken from both ends, with each part meeting in the middle down to the last millimetre, guided by a GPS. We think that electrical activity plays the role of the GPS and, at the same time, this activity modifies itself progressively, allowing the process to be followed – a kind of construction site meeting. This activity acts like a checkpoint, running continuous quality control, similarly to compliance checks in industrial production chains (see discussion in (Ben-Ari & Spitzer, 2010)). The studies that we have conducted over many decades on rodents, primates, and on prematurely born babies for certain parts confirm this sequence, its maturation, and its electric signals.

This system seeks to inform the neurons' targets as to the location and maturation stage in which the neuron finds itself. For the visual system, each ganglionic neuron in the retina, of which there are a million, lengthen towards our visual centres and send this information to their targets. A visual system builds itself from this information. It is therefore a sophisticated GPS, which can indicate space, time, location, and age all at the same time. A second function of the system is the taking into account of external conditions and adaption to these. It will do this by changing the programme if need be. Nothing is immutable; continuous control is exercised, which takes external conditions into account. Complex genetic biochemical pathways fine-tune and modify the programme's execution at every point in time. Thus, we can identify at the DNA level the regulatory genes that control the turning on or off of thousands of other genes, enabling this true strike force to totally amend the execution of a programme. These genes are turned on by other genes or by external events, the role of which is to cause a chain of events when the time comes, as well as the chance to correct or amend any given part of the programme. We will see that these genes are also often the targets of mutations that cause severe disorders like Rett syndrome, the symptoms of which are also shared by autism.

To conclude, one of the major discoveries in the study of brain maturation is the electrical language of immature neurons that differs from adult ones. The developing brain is not a little adult brain. It has its own ionic currents, discharge patterns and electrical properties. The goal of these activities is different from that of the adult brain. It does not codify information precisely and swiftly like those that enable quick responses to stimuli from the outside world or, for the blessed ones among us, that allow the playing of Bach's violin sonatas. The brain's construction is therefore built from a genetic programme, whilst also maintaining flexibility by allowing the environment to influence its execution and adaptation to conditions. The developing brain receives a lot of information generated by the periphery. The data are analysed in real time and provides the elements for the programme's functioning and adaptation. In the next chapter, we will look at an example of a maturation sequence to illustrate how the brain develops; this has been extensively investigated and used as a model for developmental sequences.

4. A maturation sequence: immature neurons are richer in chloride than adult ones

It all started when one of us, Yehezkel Ben-Ari, was named director of an INSERM unit (the French National Institute for Health and Medical Research) at the Port-Royal Maternity Hospital in 1986, taking over from Professor Alexandre Minkowski. In order to immerse ourselves at the heart of the maternity hospital, we decided to study the maturation of brain activity and the various pathologies that can afflict the brain. The first recordings we took allowed us to discover utterly unexpected properties, which were clearly difficult to place within our contemporary frameworks. The GABAergic currents clearly had properties that were totally different from adult ones. These currents were supposed to inhibit neural activity but instead excited it because of the high intracellular chloride concentrations present in immature neurons (Ben-Ari, 2014; Ben-Ari, Cherubini, Corradetti, & Gaiarsa, 1989; Ben-Ari, Gaiarsa, Tyzio, & Khazipov, 2007). The activation of a receptor causes chloride to exit rather than enter, like in adult neurons, such that the GABA then causes the rest potential to depolarise rather than hyperpolarise, often resulting in neural excitation. This observation, which has been confirmed in very many species and brain structures, seems to have been maintained throughout evolution and constitutes a major developmental property of the brain.

When chloride transporters mature

A chloride importer with a mouthful of a name, NKCC1 is among the important regulators of intracellular chloride concentrations. It allows two chloride molecules to enter in exchange for one sodium molecule (Na+) and one potassium molecule (K+). Another one also exists, a chloride exporter called KCC2 that returns the process to equilibrium. It allows two chloride molecules to exit for two potassium molecules. This mechanism ensures that the flux of chloride is controlled because it must retain a specific stability to ensure the proper functioning of neural networks. The transporter that lets the chloride in starts working before the exit transporter does, resulting in an accumulation of chloride in the nerve cell (Rivera et al., 1999). We can study the functioning and the role of these transporters thanks to molecules that prevent the selective means by which one transporter or another is blocked. Thus, a molecule like bumetanide selectively blocks NKCC1, lowering the intracellular chloride concentration and reinforcing the inhibition of young neurons. This molecule, which we will explore at length later, is a diuretic that acts at the kidney level, where NKCC1 controls diuresis. This state of affairs is not unique, indeed it is present in the brain and in peripheral organs, where a good number of proteins and transporters exercise the same functions. Intestinal motility, for example, is controlled via neuron receptors that work in this way.

What is the point of having neurons and GABA synapses that excite in the first place?

The excitation of GABA receptors in immature neurons that have high chloride concentrations is linked to an increase in intracellular calcium. This calcium, which actually exists in small concentrations when free, plays a central role as trophic factor acting on growth, the burgeoning and the formation of synapses, or cellular plasticity. Essentially, GABA first excites, taking on a trophic role, then, when the density of the glutamate synapses is high enough, the transporter that drains chloride becomes operational, changing the GABA's action polarity (Ben-Ari, 2014; Ben-Ari et al., 2007). Nature does things well. The alternative mechanism with a precise minute by minute control of the excitatory and inhibitory drives is far too rigid implying a genetic automated control of every one of the hundreds of molecules involved in synaptic operation.

What are the clinical implications of this sequence?

If GABA excites immature neurons while inhibiting adult ones, a chemical that would improve GABA's effectiveness would have an opposite effect on the brain of the mother than on the brain of the foetus. Valium® and other benzodiazepines thus have anxiolytic, soporific or anaesthetic effects in adults by increasing the inhibitive effect, while the opposite is true for the immature brain. We can easily imagine what the implications of such an observation are, especially given that many molecules are often given to pregnant women to treat insomnia and depression. The same goes for cannabis, which acts on the GABAergic synapses and can cause undesirable effects on the development of the embryo brain. Other circumstances are just as delicate. With a pregnant woman who is epileptic, for example, we seek to prevent fits during pregnancy that may cause an abortion by administering molecules that exert aberrant actions. Thus, there are antiepileptic agents that act on GABA signalling and that have been found to increase the incidence of autism in newborns, having a deleterious effect on the foetus brain development. Experimental observations provide compelling observations that blocking the high chloride levels *in utero* for instance by maternal administration of bumetanide during gestation can be toxic leading to offspring with autism (Wang & Kriegstein, 2011). These observations also underline another important aspect of the development of new medicine: a pharmacopoeia specifically dedicated to pregnant women and new born is much needed. Indeed, until recently, the molecules used to treat new born were the same as those used for adults. There was no obligation to test these molecules on young animals. Legislators have since changed tack and it is now obligatory to test molecules developed for newborns on young animals. We will see other examples later on where different treatments are necessary for developing brains.

5. Childbirth: a special highly vulnerable moment

Childbirth is a complex process during which hundreds of molecules and signalling pathways act in concert. It is in fact the most complex biological event in mammals. The goal of all these adjustments, which happen only at birth, is that of adapting to a new environment. There is, for example, the preparation of the lungs for a shift from an aquatic to an oxygenated environment, involving the reduction of water levels in the lungs but also major shifts of metabolic, cardiovascular, immune system and microbiota during this period. Birth is a very stressful event (Lagercrantz & Slotkin, 1986) with levels of stress molecules in the baby higher than anything that we shall experience in our lives. These levels are in fact much higher than the ones observed in the mother giving birth. This stress is indispensable for some of the events that must take place rapidly notably the first breath. This probably underlines the observation that following C-section delivery, there is less stress molecules but also some initial difficulty to breath. During evolution, the challenge was to both provide a system –stress molecules – that will enable the abrupt and rapid shift but also to protect brain neurons from this excessive stress. Indeed, neurons are not at ease in presence of very high levels of stress molecules being associated with enhanced excitability and even seizures produced notably by an accumulation of chloride in neurons and a shift of GABA actions from inhibition to excitation. How is it possible to reconcile these two opposite requirements?

Among the molecules involved, oxytocin appears to play a particularly important role. This hormone, which already operate to trigger uterine contractions and childbirth, also plays a key role in the mother-child relationship after birth and during breastfeeding in humans and animals. In experimental conditions when this hormone is prevented from operating, the mother is indifferent to her offspring. Indeed, there exists a close relationship between oxytocin concentrations and the sociability of certain animal species. We reasoned that perhaps it also, plays a role in the alterations of GABA polarity during birth.

During a focused study conducted on rodents recording neurons from the embryonic to the adult stage, we discovered a completely unexpected result when examining the change curve of intracellular chloride concentration (Tyzio et al., 2006). It must be admitted that we were confounded, as it did not initially make sense! That is the surprise of discovery. The curve describing the fall in chloride concentrations had an abrupt inflexion a few hours before and after birth. It was as if birth was announced by a dip in intracellular chloride concentrations in the newborn's brain. Knowing that oxytocin triggers birth, it was of course necessary to check the hypothesis that oxytocin was at the origin of this fall in chloride concentrations. The key experiment consisted in injecting a molecule that specifically blocks oxytocin's action. We were able to see that administering this molecule stops the fall in chloride in the neurons of newborn rats. In other words, the same molecule that prompts labour acts also on central neurons of the newborn, causing a diminution in chloride. Oxytocin released by the mother, or by the future baby in some species, provokes birth and at the same time acts on the newborn's brain. That is some multitasking of Swiss Army Knife proportions! This fall in chloride, the readers will have understood, means a reduction in GABA's excitatory effects in favour of increased inhibition. This translates into a reduction in central neural activity and a greater resistance to external aggressions, such as reduced oxygen levels, that are a major cause of neurological disorders.

The brutal fall in chloride during birth is hugely important. Indeed, one of the major causes of brain injuries, birth handicaps, and motor disabilities are temporary absences of oxygen called hypoxic-ischaemic episodes. They are generated by a number of factors, such as the umbilical cord contracting or poor irrigation of the brain during labour. They are even more dangerous if there are high levels of electrical or metabolic activity. These hypoxic-ischaemic episodes will translate into brain injuries that often cause neonatal epilepsy that can persist throughout life. On the other hand, oxytocin has a neuro-protective effect on the newborn's brain by inhibiting brain activity during birth (Tyzio et al., 2006). And that is not all: it also has analgesic effects, relieving pain. The initial observations were made by Dr Lagercrantz's group in Sweden, which showed that vaginal delivery babies feel less pain than C–section delivery ones (Bergqvist, Katz-Salamon, Hertegard, Anand, & Lagercrantz, 2009). The baby endures a painful process during birth and this observation suggested that oxytocin might reduce that pain. We confirmed that this is the case in rodents. The concentration of intracellular chloride in pain cells is high and reduced by the hormone while its antagonist worsens the sensation of pain in animals right after birth (Mazzuca et al., 2011). So, the hormone that triggers labour and delivery also protects the child's brain and reduces pain during childbirth. We cannot be anything but awed by Mother Nature's genius that, here as elsewhere, she uses one mechanism to solve many problems. It is not impossible that we will become increasingly interested in molecules of this type in the future when seeking to prevent dangerous effects from occurring during childbirth (Ben-Ari, 2015). Therefore, during evolution, the possible deleterious actions on neurons of stress needed for major biological functions during birth including respiration was compensated by the same hormone that triggers birth. The fact that the various actions of oxytocin are mediated by an action on chloride levels and the polarity of GABA actions reinforces the importance of this parameter that stands at the core of so many developmental and pathological issues.

Whether C-sections increase the incidence of autism has long been debated with contradictory epidemiological observations. This is quite understandable as the heterogeneity of C-sections renders difficult to conclude. C-sections can be performed because of urgency – complications and obvious evidence that the fetus suffers for one reason or another. However, the incidence of seizures has increased worldwide with over 50% in some countries (Brazil, Egypt), around 20 in others (Europe) and slightly higher in the USA. This is the result of both legal aspects with less parents suing the hospital if complications have occurred after C-section than vaginal delivery – but also "fashion" – with well-known actors having done it leading to the "why not me" mind-set' – and career – women wanting to do it rapidly and to go back to work! Earlier studies have suggested that there is no link between C-section and autism in offspring. A more recent study relying on a very large number of papers and studies suggests in contrast that there is a small but significant increase in the incidence of autism after C-section delivery. However, epidemiological investigations aren't sufficient to conclude this because of the heterogeneity of cases and the difficulty to differentiate between C-sections made in emergency and others.

We therefore decided to test the hypothesis in mice, where the conditions are well controlled and homogeneous. Interestingly, this important issue has seldom been investigated earlier with only two laboratories having adapted a surgical intervention to perform a C-section in rodents. We made several attempts to develop the technique and after a long period we succeeded to have pups elevated by a foster mother after a C-section delivery. We then used all our techniques to determine if the brain and neurons are altered in pups born by vaginal delivery and by age matched C-sections. We used both term C-sections – fetuses being removed at term by C-sections – and "preterm" C-section – where fetuses are removed 24 hours earlier. We could not remove the fetuses earlier as the lungs are not mature, but it bears stressing that the duration of gestation is 19-21 days and hence 1 day difference is a significant period (corresponding roughly to two weeks in a human pregnancy). From the electrophysiological aspect, we found no difference between term, preterm C-sections and vaginal delivery, suggesting that delivery does not impact the alterations produced by oxytocin and the abrupt shift of chloride (see above). This was also the case with a variety of behavioral features that were not altered, with the exception of calls made by the pups when separated from the mother early on, but these effects were short lasting. Also, reconstructing neurons revealed that they were slightly smaller following C-section delivery, but this difference was abolished 1 day later as if there was a delay that was corrected within 1 day. Collectively, this study suggests that C-section at least in rodents and in the short time frame possible does not impact the process, and that the brain is not affected by the lack of vaginal delivery and associated events (Fernandez et al., 2018).

Therefore, the GABA developmental shift during birth is an important signal with oxytocin playing a number of important roles as an anti-stress molecule endowed also with a neuro-protective action on metabolic insults during this vulnerable period.

6. High intracellular chloride concentrations in epilepsy and other pathological disorders: back to the future

Many brain disorders have been associated with an excess excitatory drive mediated by an imbalance between excitation and inhibition. This can be due to an increase of the former and/or a decrease of the latter. Is it possible that alterations of the GABA shift and chloride levels also operate in pathological conditions as they do during birth? Epilepsies was obviously the first type of pathology to investigate in this regard and the initial measures of the effects of pathological conditions on intracellular chloride came from studies dedicated to epilepsies. One of the most frequent brain disorders, epilepsy constitutes a large family of disorders associated with intense highly synchronized aberrant electrical activities of brain networks associated with a large panel of clinical symptoms. Studying epilepsy has helped to better understand the normal functioning of the brain and its pathological disorders. During an epileptic fit, all or some of the brain's neurons discharge their electrical signals in a synchronised manner, as opposed to the large-scale discharge patterns observed in physiological disorders. With epilepsy, the equilibrium between excitation and inhibition is disturbed and the regulation of intracellular chloride undergoes a tough ordeal. Inevitably, chloride levels were expected to increase and this indeed was found to be the case at least in many animal models of epileptic disorders. Perhaps more astonishingly, similar increases of neuronal chloride was then observed in a large panel of brain disorders extending from brain trauma, spinal cord injuries, ischemic insults, Parkinson disease, chronic pain, Post-Traumatic Stress Disorders (PTSD), developmental disorders and even certain types of carcinogenic tumours (Ben-Ari, 2017).

These observations have important clinical implications. Let's look at an example: a good number of antiepileptic molecules act by improving the efficiency of GABA currents. Since they allow chloride to enter and end up controlling the amplitude of the currents generated by the GABAergic synapses, they end up facilitating cerebral inhibition. Many of these molecules are known to the non-scientific public, such as barbiturates and benzodiazepines (of which Valium® is well-known). Beyond their antiepileptic effect, they also act as anaesthetic, anxiolytic or even analgesic agents. Nevertheless, if GABA excites neurons notably because of high neuronal levels of chloride, these agents will have different or even opposite effects to those they would have in healthy tissue. Thus, as we have seen, Valium® will inhibit neurons in pregnant women, while exciting those in the embryo. If GABA excites neurons rather than inhibiting them, however, these same products can logically have paradoxical pro-epileptic effects and worsen fits!

Many clinical and experimental observations corroborate these paradoxical effects. Furthermore, they show that the paradoxical effects are more important than the fits that happen before the phenobarbital is administered, suggesting that the recurrence of fits produces an increasingly acute accumulation of chloride. This is because chloride concentrations become more difficult to regulate when there is a recurrence of fits. When experiments are conducted, the phenobarbital reduces the number of early fits but worsens those that occur later on. Therefore, the effectiveness of antiepileptic medication is determined by the *timing* of when it is administered. New therapeutic solutions might therefore be possible if chloride concentrations were to be reduced back to their original levels, thereby restoring GABA's hyperpolarising and inhibitory action.

It is from these indirect observations that our hypothesis of reducing chloride concentrations with a diuretic was born. The diuretic would increase the efficiency of antiepileptic molecules acting on GABA. Indeed, NKCC1, the co-transporter we looked at previously, is one of the main importers of chloride into the kidneys. It controls the removal of water *by* transporting chloride. However, this very same importer of chloride is also present in the brain and is expressed during embryogenesis, being, as we have seen, one of the factors responsible for high chloride concentrations in immature neurons. We quickly came to the conclusion that a diuretic decreases chloride concentrations in epileptic rodents' neurons and thus improves the efficiency of GABAergic inhibition. Admittedly, similar changes were observed in some but not all models of epilepsies. In addition, things became more complex when we and others discovered that recurrent seizures acutely increase neuronal chloride suggesting that seizures might beget more seizures by this mechanism, hence the difficulty to generalize the putative efficacy of reducing chloride to all types of epilepsies. An extra complication came from our observations that recurrent seizures generated in a given brain structure can propagate to distal regions leading there to the formation of an epileptic focus. An additional blow came from a small clinical trial on two-days-old babies in Europe who suffered from severe neonatal anoxic seizures. The trial had to be stopped because side effects on the auditory system. This might however have been anticipated considering the susceptibility of the developing hearing system to a mixture of antibiotics and diuretics. Two lessons from these studies may be gleaned: first, the diuretic might raise concerns when applied early in life in particular in conditions where antibiotics are required, and second recurrent seizures have an impact on chloride regulation and the effectiveness of the diuretic might depend on the number of seizures that occur prior to the administration. In addition, using this drug during pregnancy might raise severe concerns.

Following that, and as is often the case in science, we and many other laboratories found that the changes in intracellular chloride concentrations did not only concern epilepsy: other pathologies were also characterised by an accumulation of chloride in neurons. These pathologies include brain injuries, as well as bone marrow injuries, brain trauma or chronic bone pain, and are linked to an increase in intracellular chloride and GABA's excitatory effects. There seems to be a kind of general response to aggressions or brain injuries: a deficient chloride regulation system, a reorganisation of the circuits and the expression of currents and signals usually characteristic of a brain in formation. Why such a variety of insults lead to some common alterations remains a mystery. This is also corroborated by the observation that drugs to develop a given disorder are also often found to be efficient for other ones, raising the possibility that common mechanisms might operate perhaps in relation with at least some of the clinical manifestations in relation with general neuronal excitability that these drugs reduce. These observations are what led us to propose treating autism with a diuretic. Gaining compelling experimental data took a few years but astonishingly they were preceded rather than as usual followed by clinical trials.

II

What is Autism and Related Disorders?

Autism is a neurodevelopmental condition affecting one child in 59 and more than 2% of boys, according to the latest figures from the US Centre for Disease Control (Baio et al., 2018). It is a developmental disorder that impacts three principal areas: social relations, communication, and behaviour. We can define autism simply as the absence of a social instinct that characterises people who have a 'normal' development, generally described as 'neurotypical'. Autism was first described by two doctors who did not know each other but who depicted the well-known triad of autism with a single year separating them. Kanner wrote about it in English in 1943, whilst Asperger published his observations in German in 1944 but was only recognised for his contribution in the 1980s when translated in English by Lorna Wing. The cases he described related to children who had normal language acquisition, and behaved like "little professor", and could be very gifted. Incidentally, she regretted later this publicity that was undue because Asperger appeared to have been a convinced Nazi, in favour of forced sterilisation of unfit persons and who sent many children to death, being not suitable for the 'glorious' society planned by the Fuhrer (Czech, 2018). On the other hand, it is possible that Asperger wanted to avoid labelling these children as 'mentally retarded', which would have had them sent to concentration camps. In any case, 'high-functioning autism' can be used as an alternative term for Asperger syndrome, although many high-functioning autistic individuals do like to refer to themselves as "Aspies", and there is some important value in that diagnosis for those affected (Attwood, 2007), and even if obviously there is no way to defend whatever Hans Asperger did during WWII, he still seems to have first described this syndrome.

It was only in the 1980s that DSM-III, the psychiatrists' bible, finally recognised autism as a category in itself rather than a psychosis (Pichot, 1986). Later, the DSM-IV defined categories within ASD comprising of Autistic Disorder, Pervasive Developmental Disorders, Not Otherwise Specified (PDD NOS), Asperger's Disorder, Rett Disorder and Childhood Disintegrative Disorders. This was then revised in the 2013 DSM-5 which define one broad category "Autism Spectrum Disorder", that then needs to be specified in terms of the presence or absence of intellectual impairment, language impairment, the presence of a known medical or genetic condition or environmental factor, and the association with another neurodevelopmental, mental or behavioural disorder, and Asperger syndrome is no longer a separate category in the DSM-5.

What is most striking about autism is its incredible variety of clinical forms and the fact that we use the same term to qualify people who have pronounced intellectual disability, people who cannot speak, those who display self-mutilating behaviour, and others who subscribe to the triad but who have a normal if not above-average level of intelligence. That is why we prefer to speak of an autism spectrum, or of the autisms (Coleman & Gillberg, 2012), rather than simply of 'autism'.

When it comes to genetics, it has been clearly established that individuals are five to ten times more likely to be autistic when they have a sibling who is autistic. It has also been shown that there is a 70 to 90% concordance between identical twins. Some families are more prone than others to exhibit autistic traits, suggesting that heredity plays an important role. Ever since the pioneering study by a group of French scientists that identified a mutation in a Swedish family, hundreds of mutations that correlate with an autistic syndrome have been identified. Each mutation may only be relevant to a handful of individuals on the planet, others may affect between 0.1 and 1% of people, with the total number of mutations estimated to be relevant to roughly 15 to 20% of autistic people. But there remains a huge majority of afflicted individuals who are without a mutation. Furthermore, the same mutation in two brothers may produce two totally different clinical situations, with the first exhibiting severe autism, including a lack of speech, and the second being diagnosed with high-functioning Asperger's. Technology has allowed the search for the loophole in the huge genetic alphabet to be undertaken speedily and with costs divided by a thousand. From this starting point, geneticists have now postulated that all those with autism have the same mutation or even that there is a master gene that triggers the disorder and that it is simply a question of time as to when we will locate it. The issue is that, in science, it is not possible to extrapolate therapy from a single principle. To say that autism is a 'genetic' disorder is an abuse of language, unless we decide that the weak percentage of autistic people who have a mutation represent the majority. Recent studies however provide a vivid illustration with the progressively emerging observations that genes are controlled by epigenetic factors that provide a link between genes and environment. In essence, the idea is that genes are not *Deus ex Machina* switches that trigger on their own disorders, but that they are controlled by many factors, including peripheral and environmental ones. These factors trigger common switches capable of activating or inactivating a single or a plethora of genes. Viewed from this perspective, genes share with many other messengers the capacity of modifying ongoing activity and brain function. Modifications of these switch control devices has been shown to operate in many disorders including autism. Collectively, these observations shed more acute light on the complex routes followed by an insult to produce a disorder.

To conclude, a single gene defect does not underlie a disorder as complex as autism. It is possible that the combination of tens or hundreds of mutations can be clearly translated into autism but it is difficult to see how this will lead to treatments. Yet, this reductionist approach ignores the fundamental role played by the environment and by brain activity in modulating brain formation and the dynamic consequences of the mutation on brain construction. It is crucial to determine how genes and environment interact if we are to appreciate and one day cure this syndrome, bearing in mind its *in utero* origins and characteristic communication deficiencies. In addition, the neuro-archeology concept that posits that intrauterine insults deviate developmental sequences suggests that the modifications produced by the pathogenic trigger are the real cause of the disease and the one amenable to treatment when the diagnosis is made (often several years later). We shall return to the conceptual aspects of this debate later on.

III

A New Treatment for Autism?

1. A meeting and strange ideas

Illnesses in children are always unbearable, and even more so when we are powerless in proposing a therapy for it. It induces a tenacious will to fight, to give all in order to share with others their pain and feelings of injustice. Parents and loved ones do not hold back in their efforts to remain together on the lookout for anything that could improve the daily lives of their children. This translates into the founding of associations for autistic individuals. These are powerful lobbies that continually remind politicians, researchers, doctors, and other key figures of their duties. They are a means for this energy to express itself, for pain and information to be channelled. Even if their actions sometimes err in an unfavourable direction, it is never due to bad intentions. Truthfully, it is often such associations that actually make things happen. And the volunteers involved are no more gullible than Saint Thomas of Aquinas, they will not just take whatever is said as truth. Researchers and clinicians quickly realise that miraculous solutions will not do.

The many associations focusing on autism in France, such as *Vaincre l'autisme*, ARAPI, and *Autism France*, may be in competition but are always unified in their goals. *Vaincre l'autisme* is an association that organises an important meeting in Paris each year, whilst ARAPI enlivens its members during autumn schools held every two years in Le Croisic, Britanny. They are information-sharing gatherings during which researchers, health workers, and educators present technological and scientific innovations within the beautiful setting of an ancient building overlooking the Opal Sea. There, discussions are pervaded by the aroma of the Atlantic that is so distinct to a Mediterranean like Y. Ben-Ari.

Basic research is sometimes accused of being too far from daily life, of being impractical (the holy profitability of a world subjugated to the goddess Productivity and her mother, Growth). Basic researchers also happily tell psychiatrists off for not being more interested in hard science when dealing with the question of how to relieve patients, clinicians being by default engaged in applied research. Researchers and clinicians find themselves in the same situation as the polar bear and the whale that haunt the same places without ever meeting (to borrow Daniel Widlöcher's parable), when it is by meeting that new perspectives are germinated.

The fruitful merit of these meetings is that basic scientists are facing clinicians and more importantly parents of children with autism reminding them the urgency of finding a cure. The president of ARAPI invited Yehezkel Ben-Ari to speak at one of the association's autumn schools about brain development and disorders. Dr Éric Lemonnier, a clinician convinced by the poverty of present concepts of how the disorder emerges and its neurodevelopmental roots is present and struck by Ben-Ari's conference. At the end of the presentation, Yehezkel Ben-Ari explained that, because of the maturation of GABA neurons, the agonistic effect (which reinforces GABA's action) is inversed in the adults and in the foetus: 'If we were to give a pregnant woman Valium®, she would become subdued, whereas the foetus would become excited.' Dr Lemonnier's clinical experience had taught him that Valium® may evoke in some autistic children a paradoxical reaction: they become excited and hyper-agitated. Parents are the ones who end up informing clinicians of this effect, which they notice when their child is given a sedative during a medical exam, such as when going to the dentist. A publication, which was deemed anecdotal at the time, similarly confirmed this observation. The link albeit very indirect and far from being demonstrated became one on which to rely, and history could begin.

If these children presented a paradoxical reaction to GABA's agonists, it was maybe because the neurons were excitatory, due to high intracellular chloride concentrations as experimental data suggests. If we reduced these concentrations, the neurons would then become inhibitory, as in most people. At this point in our thought process, we had scant knowledge of the clinical translation from excitatory to inhibitory neurons. We were simply led by the idea that being able to intervene at the neurodevelopmental stage might enable a translation in some of the maturation processes particular to autistic people (such as neuro-sensorial and psycho-cognitive processes). As we have previously seen, the transportation of chloride into the cell is managed by NKCC1 and out of the cell by KCC2. When researchers want to inhibit NKCC1 during an *in vitro* experiment, they use bumetanide. The choice of treatment for reducing the intracellular chloride concentrations in the GABA neurons was before us. Bumetanide is a diuretic identified by Feit in 1971. It has been used in adults to treat arterial hypertension and in newborns to reduce an oedema. We therefore had good knowledge of the diuretic effect, potential side effects and the supervision required when it is prescribed. Yet two key questions remained: what posology was needed and how to measure the treatment's benefits?

As to the posology, we established that we must stay with small doses as bumetanide would stop acting solely on NKCC1 at higher ones, it would instead start affecting other transporters, risking a loss of efficiency or other undesirable effects. Side effects are also more likely to occur with a higher posology. When bumetanide is used in infants to reduce an oedema, the doses range from 0.1 mg/kg to 0.3 mg/kg. We concluded that 0.5 mg would be suitable for children of three years of age and higher. The half-life of bumetanide (time taken by an organism to eliminate half of the chemical initially present) is around an hour and a half (it varies from patient to patient but remains rather short). We therefore decided to propose a treatment made up of two daily doses of 0.5 mg, one in the morning and one in the evening (Lemonnier & Ben-Ari, 2010). The clinical trials would be undertaken with children aged between three and eleven years old. Why did we not adapt the posology according to the child's weight? This question is actually relevant to every psychotropic prescription for children. A treatment for which we seek a peripheral action (that is, one outside the central nervous system) must of course be adapted to the child's weight. However, when we need an action to take place in the brain and when the blood-brain barrier depends on a transporter rather than blood levels, adapting dosage to body weight is more complex. Selective Serotonin Recapture Inhibitors (SSRIs) are thus used in the same doses whether it is in children or in adults.

Yet, at this stage, these ideas were largely conjectural as the paradoxical actions of Valium® were not necessarily due to elevated neuronal chloride, that anyhow had not been demonstrated in animal models of autism. In addition, a considerable complication stemmed from the fact that the life time of bumetanide – the time it takes to be degraded and thus ineffective- are short, at best a few hours. Also, perhaps more problematic, bumetanide does not cross easily the Blood Brain Barrier – a barrier that protects the brain from unwanted molecules. It is thus quite difficult to explain how a short-lived molecule that in addition does not readily penetrate the brain can exert its positive actions on the brain. In this kind of situations, the scientist is left with two possibilities: rejecting the concept and utility of performing clinical trials, or adopt a transitory philosophy, gathering clinical and experimental observations to check if the hypothesis is still valid. In that case, either novel data would provide other explanations or invalidate the observations that suggest poor brain penetrability at least in pathological conditions. We decided to use this alternative reasoning: if the drug attenuated autism, this would already be an achievement, and perhaps alternative explanations would later pop out.

The other question was how to measure a therapeutic effect. A number of clinical scales have been developed for autism. The oldest is the *Childhood Autism Rating Scale* (CARS), which focuses on autism's symptoms evaluated by the treating psychiatrist. It looks at fifteen items, thirteen of which are to do with autism symptoms. Of the last two, one measures intellectual level and the other is based on the clinician's opinion. The scale ranks the intensity of the disorder and has been employed in diagnosis for a long time. The development of other diagnostic scales (*Autism Diagnostic Interview*, or ADI-R, and *Autism Diagnostic Observation Schedule*, or ADOS), which are better adapted to the classification systems used today (DSM-V and CIM-10) have rendered CARS mostly redundant. Most of the work done on evaluating different treatments for autism use the *Autism Behavior Checklist* (ABC), which is a non-specific scale that measures the expressions of the disorder's challenge of adapting to everyday life (these expressions include reactions like aggressiveness, agitation, and so on). The treatments most frequently used for autism are atypical antipsychotics, which target the specific behavioural expressions. Evaluating the efficiency of these treatments is successful when we use ABC, whilst CARS is often inadequate for measuring the effect. Indeed, CARS is now little used and has gained a reputation for being poorly-adapted to measuring therapeutic effects. Other measures are better suited and indeed more frequently used. Thus, Social Responsive Scale (SRS) is a large scale (over 60 parameters) estimated by the parents – not the treating psychiatrist – who are asked to fill questionnaires weekly reporting the changes that they see. An amelioration by 10 points of SRS is considered by the FDA as being sufficient to claim a positive action of a drug on autism. Interestingly, SRS is considered more reliable than CARS in the US but not in Europe, denoting a preferred reliability on parents in the former and psychiatrists than in the latter. These debates are important as the placebo effect is a major issue in evaluating positive treatments in particular as far as autism in children is considered. There is no simple answer to the question of the best way of determining the actions of a drug on a complex disorder. We were also faced with the issue of inclusion parameters, were we to only accept say adolescents with high functioning autism (Asperger's)? Children without seizures? Relying on IQ measures? As we had no idea on which parameters or age or autism type, the drug might be beneficial, we adopted an equilibrated position of not selecting according to age or severity but only to exclude epilepsies – as an attenuation of seizures recurrence might be confounded with amelioration of the core symptoms of autism and with no additional drugs treatment as the results whether positive or negative might be ascribed to the combination of effects. We also decided to use CARS that seemed better adapted to our initial goals of determining the effects of bumetanide on certain core symptoms of autism, rather than on the behavioural disorders associated with autism. The diagnostic scales, not developed to measure the intensity of the disorders, seemed to us less adapted, especially given that the therapeutic trial was to last for three months. For this reason, determining the IQ and the actions of the treatment on IQ was not considered reliable, as this is a parameter difficult to determine in 3 years old children and a change in IQ in 3 months is unlikely.

When it comes to proving the benefits of a treatment, medicine has rigorous methods. Only controlled and random double-blind studies are employed (where neither the patient nor the doctor know whether the substance administered is an active compound or a placebo). When statistical tests are applied, we accept that there is a 5% risk of being wrong (that is, we accept that in 5% of cases we will wrongly find a therapeutic effect). Proving a therapeutic effect will therefore have to be confirmed by trials in other centres (repetition reduces the risk of being wrong).

We developed a therapeutic study with the Brest CHRU's clinical investigation centre and obtained authorisation for the trial from the relevant people protection committee and health product monitoring agency. The cost involved was large and we first sought funding from hospital clinical research programmes. We were unsuccessful and it seemed to us that a preliminary open study on five patients would help us obtain the necessary financial support. This open study would also allow us to validate our choice regarding posology and clinical scale. The first five patients made up a voluntarily heterogeneous group of autistic children. The heterogeneity had to do with their age (three to eleven years old) and their developmental characteristics (from pronounced developmental delay, where one eleven-year-old had a developmental age of eleven months, to no delay at all). From a strictly diagnostic standpoint, we sought to limit our trials only to children who matched the diagnosis of infantile autism and to Asperger's syndrome. Indeed, it was important to us to evaluate the treatment in different progressive forms of autism, which made it essential for us not to homogenise the population studied but to take a small representative sample of the various forms and severities of the spectrum. These five children therefore took 0.5 mg of bumetanide morning and night for three months. The clinical evaluation depended on CARS (which we established by speaking with the parents, filming the child while they were engaged in a communication exchange, and using the ADOS protocol, which allowed us to create the same situation at the start and after three months). We also used the ABC, the *Clinical Global Impression* scale, and scales developed in Tours, France. This enabled us to see which symptoms were being acted on by the treatment and whether the scales usually used in therapeutic trials for autism were the right ones. The results were positive in all five patients for all the scales employed. But this was not enough to obtain the financing. Then, the CHRU of Brest decided to cut costs and both clinical research directors and the clinical investigation centre had to give up all remuneration for their work. We thus started the trial using funding that we raised ourselves (as we will see later).

This second trial (Lemonnier et al., 2012) included sixty patients with autism and Asperger's aged between three and twelve years. Half of them received a placebo while others took bumetanide. Neither the patients, the parents, nor the clinicians knew who had taken which. The results showed a significantly positive effect on CARS and on the CGI scale, whilst the other scales showed little significant improvement. The difference between this result and that of the first experiment on the five patients is due to the difference between an open study, where each knows what they take, and a double-blind, randomised trial that is more sensitive to the placebo effect. Improving CARS taught us that bumetanide acts at the heart of autism's symptoms. Strict medical monitoring must accompany the prescription in case of side effects (which are inherent to any treatment). Indeed, a quarter of patients exhibited hypokalaemia, which is easily dealt with by potassium supplements. To this day, we have not observed any other unexpected side effects, except of course diuresis, hypokalaemia, and related ones like fatigue or, rarely, anorexia. At the end of the three months of treatment, an extra month was dedicated to being monitored without any treatment being administered so that any latent side effects could be recorded. None were observed. All the parents asked that their child return to the open treatment, with some convinced that this month-long period was accompanied by a loss of the therapeutic effect, whilst others had met parents of a child who had been treated. Even if generally positive, exchanges between parents can create a risk that the prescription of a treatment is deemed generally successful, when proof of its overall effectiveness has yet to be fully established. One example of this was when a child, a few years ago, started to speak after a therapeutic trial with secretin. The next day, TV stations broadcasted the news and, six months later, more than four thousand children were taking secretin despite any further proof of its effectiveness. Double-blind studies later revealed no effectiveness and people stopped taking secretin altogether. In our case, the positive results obtained from the double-blind study constituted important proof, though it needed to be reproduced by other teams. With all these precautions, we were able to conclude a lack of side effects other than hypokalaemia (with some patients observing from four years' hindsight) and, importantly, improvement that reinforced with time. Some 'high-functioning' autism patients noted that their child was getting more excited towards the end of the morning and that this would stop when the afternoon dose was taken. Parents proposed taking the dose towards the end of the morning when possible, but we observed that the excitation returned at the end of the afternoon. The short half-life of bumetanide means that it must either be taken more often or that the dosage must be increased. Multiplying the number of intakes is sometimes not easy to fit into the daily lives of these children. We therefore opted for increasing the dosage to 1 mg in the morning and at the end of the afternoon, which led to a more tangible clinical result. There was a consequent increase in the number of patients with hypokalaemia, with a third of patients being affected. It must be noted that this posology has therapeutic effects in both children and adults. Bumetanide, however, seemed unsuccessful in around 25% of patients. Either this was due to a true lack of effectiveness, or we did not allow for enough time to observe the therapeutic effects in some patients. It could also be that when patients have more complex disorders, with an interplay of autism, intellectual disability, and genetic syndromes, their autistic symptomology does not respond to the same approaches.

In essence, one of the criticisms was that relying on one center can be misleading, as the effects must be confirmed by independent experts operating ion different centers. In addition, the European Medicine Association (EMA) that determines and validates the efficacy of treatments requires a dose-dependent study as well as more pharmacokinetic trials in order to better comprehend the optimal dose and associated side effects. We therefore raised the funds required to perform a completely independent trial in 8 centers in France relying on an external Contract Research Organization (CRO) – a recognized body that controls and validates trials. Our 3rd trial (Lemonnier et al., 2017) was multi-centric involving 8 French centres and 74 children, 2-18 years old – a wide range because this was a requirement of the EMA to include the entire pediatric group. The inclusion criteria were very stringent, excluding children taking another treatment – except melatonin – and having other major clinical problems notably recurrent seizures, as the positive effects of the drug might have been confounded with an antiepileptic action that bumetanide also has. Admittedly this was a difficult decision, but we trusted an essential one if we wanted to ensure a genuine link between treatment and ASD attenuation. We selected 8 French centers endowed with both clinical experience in treating children with ASD and at least some experience in participating in clinical trials. The children received either bumetanide (0.5, 1 or 2 mg twice daily) or placebo, both provided as syrup with similar taste and visual presentation. To avoid or at least reduce the confounding factor of the diuresis –that occurs in bumetanide but not in placebo – the treating doctor that checked the clinical conditions and made the prescription was independent from the psychiatrist determining the alterations of the ASD. We relied on both a psychiatrist evaluation and a parental one.

The effects were statistically clear cut with in particular an amelioration of the social interactions and reduction of the agitation and repetitive behavior. This was also in accord with the observed attenuation of these parameters reported in the previous trial and in the testimony and statements of the parents both within the trial and when used outside coordinated trials. Indeed, hundreds of mails and testimonies obtained during that period from parents all over the world attested to an increased presence and attenuation of social communication deficits. Parallel trials pilot or larger trials in China and Holland confirmed the effects – they are not restricted for some mysterious reason to French population. In addition, the testimony from parents quite all over the world confirm the importance of our approach as many doctors in many countries have started to use that drug in their patients.

An additional important issue concerns the drop-out rates. In a clinical trial, any child going to a doctor or to the hospital for any reason is automatically excluded from the trial. Thus, in our second trial, children were excluded because of a ski accident, fever or other conditions. The ones relevant to the trial concerned primarily hypokalaemia and dehydration and led to a significant drop out with the highest doses (2mg twice daily) in particular in the youngest children. Thus, there was respectively no drop out with 0.5mg (twice daily), 4 drop outs (of 23) with 1mg (twice daily) and 9 (out of 22) with 2mg (twice daily). As the dosage was blindly determined, this parameter could not be controlled but suggested clearly that the highest dosage cannot be used. Interestingly, all other biological parameters including blood pressure, routine laboratory tests and hearing were not affected by the treatment as well as kidney ultrasound. Hypokalemia was as expected the most frequent adverse parameter with either mild (3 to 3.5mM/litter) or moderate (2.5 to 3mM/litter Potassium). They were treated with potassium gluconate that restored physiological blood levels.

Therefore, collectively, these observations confirm and validate the potential usefulness of bumetanide to treat autism and provide a useful basis for the dosage and conditions required to test its actions. They provide more than a proof of concept suggesting that further investment in this direction is warranted.

Although clinical authorities and psychiatry experts requires well established group data and objective criteria that can be compared in various trials, single-subject research (studies that use just one case) is useful to better understand the alterations occurring with treatment. The treating psychiatrist, like the environment of the child, also has a say as the aims of a treatment is judged at the end of the day by the extent of reintegration of the child at school and more generally in society. There are criteria that cannot be mathematically quantified requiring a more qualitative estimation of the changes. Although this does not and will not suffice to put a drug in the market for treatment, when it converges with the more classical approach, it provides a significant jump in our evaluation of the actions of the drug. A fact that seems to be well-established for the whole population does not necessarily apply systematically. It is a counter-proof, an exception that weakens the rule. The single-subject illustrates work undertaken in a population and it is with this in mind that we will move on to report some clinical cases described by Dr Lemonnier who has undoubtedly the biggest experience of treating children with bumetanide.

2. Louis and his father

Louis is three years and eight months old when his parents arrived at the Brittany autism resource centre. He has a younger brother who does not have any disorders. Louis seems happy (he is almost always smiling). I only lock eyes with him at the very start of our meeting, when I go to fetch him and his parents from the waiting room. I am crouched down to his height, calling him, and his parents say ‘Look, Louis, the doctor is coming to fetch us.’ The consultation takes place without Louis seeming to pay attention to the different people speaking to him. He prefers to play with the toys that are there at his disposal. He plays in quite a specific way, using them without building a scenario as he goes along. He just rolls the little cars, placing them at the top of a parking lot and becomes delighted when they swiftly roll down the access ramp. All seemed to go well during his first year; he was breastfed for a few months then, as his mother returned to work, his maternal grandmother and a nanny took turns taking care of him. He was a calm and observant baby who did not have any problems. He learned to walk at twelve months and started speaking early. His first words were uttered at seventeen months and were followed almost immediately by sentences at eighteen months. Despite often being silent, he speaks pretty well when he does talk.

At twenty months, his parents started getting worried because he seemed to be exhibiting a kind of regression. Eye contact was becoming rare and he would become so absorbed in activities that he would rarely respond when called; but it was his angry outbursts, when he would resist against being held by his mother and when opposition and disagreement seemed magnified, that definitively alerted the parents to the fact that something was wrong. 'He would put his hands on his ears as if he did not want to hear us.' He would go up the stairs touching each bar of the banister, and would double back to start over if he missed one; he sometimes played with his stool. Sometimes, he would be totally absorbed by the drum of the washing machine but the sound when the machine rang at the end of the cycle would be unbearable for him.

Child psychiatrists who were consulted spoke of autism and the parents therefore headed to the autism resource centre where I give the same opinion and proposed for Louis to undergo an evaluation to confirm this. The evaluation lasts two days and is made up of a series of consultations with an educator, a psychomotor therapist, a speech therapist, a psychologist, a paediatrician, a paediatric neurologist, and a geneticist. These observations not only allow us to hone in on the child's competencies and difficulties in various areas of development, they also provide shared clinical observations. The assessment is completed by undergoing an ADI-R (a conversation with the parents that investigates the symptoms of pervasive developmental disorders by observing the family during their daily life) and ADOS (a session of games and exchanges following an established sequence during which symptoms are observed). Tests are carried out to explore causative relationships and any associated disorders. These include an electroencephalogram, a brain MRI scan, a metabolic profile, a karyotype to test for Fragile X, and specific genetic searches for morpho-clinical warning signs. Following this survey, we return to the parents to update them. It is a useful moment, when we can go beyond strict diagnosis. We discuss how very early neurodevelopmental anomalies lead to specific maturations that then translate into specific cognitive processes and from which the child's behaviour ensues. At the end of this meeting, the father, brimming with wit, laughingly comments that he has the same difficulties. Sometimes it is the mothers who will say this of their husbands and when we seek to explore where the similarity lies, we find that indeed there are some relevant daily behavioural patterns but usually not the lump sum of the symptoms that lead to a specific diagnosis. Here, it is the father who, finding the explanations enlightening as to his own difficulties, asks whether he may also undergo a diagnostic evaluation. And during this exchange, Louis's mother laughs as well, saying it is her own father who is worse!

Louis's evaluation finished just as we carried out the double-blind study, so I proposed to his parents that he participate in it and they accepted. After the trial's three months were up, a month-long washout period followed and Louis's parents wanted bumetanide to be prescribed for him. Louis's participation in the therapeutic trial finished before the end of the study (it took us a while to recruit sixty patients) and so we only learned later that Louis had been administered a placebo. Throughout the time it took us to find out, however, he took the bumetanide – and this for several months. The news does not surprise the parents. Since he has started the treatment, Louis is progressing well. From the first months of taking the bumetanide, the parents noted that he was more present, that direct contact is more frequent, and that he holds gazes readily. He plays more spontaneously with other children during recess and speaks more easily. We observe, as time goes by, periods when things seem to stagnate, whilst other times show marked progress. Pain perception normalises itself: Louis, being in pain like other children after a fall or a shock, complains systematically (which he did not do previously). After eighteen months of the treatment, sounds that used to cause him distress are now easily accepted. Like all diuretic treatments, bumetanide requires strict medical and blood monitoring. Louis exhibited a fall in potassium so potassium syrup was prescribed as a supplement. He is still followed by a team of child psychologists, though this has been reduced over time. He is also schooled in a regular classroom and followed by paraprofessionals. Teachers say he is a pleasant pupil, alive and with a very good academic record. Very recently, at the end of a follow-up consultation, his mother said that he is as difficult as always to withdraw from an activity he is engaged in, though he is now interested in a greater number of things. This diversification of interests is sometimes observed when children progress in traditional schooling, so it is difficult to say whether it is due to the treatment or not. His exclusive focus makes him impervious to environmental stimuli but it usually takes 22 months or more for changes with respect to this characteristic to be observed.

A few months after Louis started the treatment, an evaluation confirmed that the father has Asperger's. He then asked us whether he may also undertake the treatment. At this point, the double-blind trial is done and the results were positive. The first functional MRI results were also positive, and so, noting the benefits the young patients were reaping from the treatment, he was prescribed bumetanide. Here are a few testimonies that he shared on the online forum of one of the Finistère associations (*Asperansa*) following his treatment:

'On my end, the treatment started last week, on Tuesday. It has been eight days. I feel well despite the complicated things happening in my life at the moment. But it is not an antidepressant. It is funny how everyone around me asks me whether I 'feel something'. It seems like they are waiting for a miracle. So I will speak frankly: I have not seen the divine light. I have not had a revelation. I need to wait at least one month before I can perhaps see a change in attitude, in behaviour… And it will first be a feeling, probably without any a real change in my behaviour. But from the first days, yes, it is better with the treatment. Better with regards to what? Why? How? I could not tell you. But I feel that it is better. I feel calmer when facing the world, when facing difficulties. Perpetual stress and anxiety when faced with a task and when dealing with how time passes, the fear of never having enough time to do things just because another must be done after and that I must prepare for it… All that seemed to be erased from the first days of the treatment.

I had a meeting this afternoon. My son was at home and I had to take care of him. Just a while ago, I would have spent all morning pacing around, waiting for the taxi booked for 1pm… But this morning, without thinking, I did the laundry, the dishes, vacuum-cleaned, played with my son, and prepared dinner.

It may not be much but I feel well. And so, I don't know… I just do things. Ernestine is surprised. Me, I do them without thinking, it seems normal to me. But three weeks ago, I would have been anxious about everything and I would not have done that. I know it well. So what are my first thought on these initial attitudes that 'do not seem like me'?… I have become a househusband.'

The next day, most of the mothers reading this testimony ask themselves whether it might not be worth obtaining such a prescription for their husbands (the housework pill).

Later, another testimony: 'Change is slow and it is difficult to be conclusive as to improvements when the treatment is still on going. But experience shows that, when it comes to the diminution of the treatment or stopping it, signs of autism that had disappeared return in spades. I now completely rule out ever stopping. I finally live full days. Gone are the wanderings, the stress, the pacing around the house without daring to do anything all morning just because I have something planned in the afternoon (school outing, work…)!

This morning, I brought the little one to school, had breakfast once I had returned, read my emails, and hunted down all the papers that I needed for an administrative file I was preparing (I'll speak about it later). I then went to the bank to ask for an appointment to open an account next week. I took the bus on the way back, had some lunch and cleaned up around the house, made myself presentable (this does not require much) and went to work. Everything was stress-free. It would have been impossible not long ago. I also noticed something particular. There are many reasons why I have not been able to look at people. During a conversation, it helps when focusing on one's thoughts without being disturbed by one's environment. It helps to concentrate on the discussion without drifting off with other thoughts. Avoiding eye contact is also sometimes a way to avoid a discomfort that is often present in men but that I cannot completely pinpoint. Sometimes it is because they, usually a woman, have sparkling eyes. Usually when they have light eyes. Eyes that dazzle… That are very disagreeable. The director of the school that my son attends was one of these women. I say 'was' because, now, I can look at her. Before, all that I knew of her was that her mouth was long and thin, her teeth white and that she smiled (nicely). The days when she was in charge, she would wear glasses. That would be too much for me, I could not even look. This is not the case anymore, for her or anyone else. (And frankly, for the school director, that is welcome as she has beautiful eyes!) I can look people in the eyes without fear of being overwhelmed. I have not yet developed the reflex, but people who know me have commented that I have started to make eye contact. My colleagues have also told me that I have changed, but they cannot say with regards to what. They only say: 'You're doing better now.' Another thing is that I can feel when it is time for me to take my medicine. I wouldn't be able to tell you how, but I feel like it is time. It is a bit like feeling short of energy, a difficulty to stay connected let us say. I have a tendency to get lost in my thoughts, a difficulty to concentrate. I take 1 mg of the bumetanide in the morning and 1 mg around 4-5pm, depending on how I feel. I did feel very tired again for the first two or three days, when I had taken the first dose, but that feeling was quickly gone. Fleeting side effects, it seems. [Note added to the testimony: we finally decided on a different dose, with 0.5 mg morning, noon and night.] There. I had regained control of my life. I could make decisions. I am much more relaxed and calm… And it seems that I have started to open myself up to others. People have told me this, without them knowing that I have Asperger's or that I have started a bumetanide treatment. Me, who thought that I was actually open and accessible! Naturally I was surprised to hear that, actually, people thought me not so much so.'

Then, after several months without participating in the forum, he wrote again: 'I have stopped because, after having difficulty accepting the diagnosis (which I had been quite certain about even before receiving the evaluation, even if I had rebuffed it as much as possible), I find that today, it is not that I have accepted the truth about who I am, it is more that I have begun to claim it. My personal experience, what I have lived through, is at the heart of my decision to stop the treatment. My son does not have thirty years' experience of living with Asperger's and so he continues the treatment. Everyone seems happy with the effects, so there is no reason to stop. Personally, I note that he is showing less pronounced, less invasive, less stressful attention to the subjects that interest him (biology and, to a lesser degree, astronomy). He does not spend all his time thinking and asking existential questions. His occupations are varied and he adapts to the relationships he develops with children his own age. Unfortunately, he still has a mindset where he will pursue what he wants and a tendency to respond to scolding with a large smile and sometimes laughter… but well… He has his father's phlegmatic personality, I can't reproach him that. All this falls in favour of the treatment.'

Around a year after starting the treatment, the father decided to stop it. When we asked him why, his reply was obvious: 'I was slower intellectually.' This man has an above-average cognitive ability (at least, as reflected by an IQ test). The exclusive sequential treatment, dedicated to Asperger's and autistic patients, is very fast in such patients (one of the patients explained that for him, the simultaneous treatment of information is of the order of the 'rapid sequential treatment'). This does not always hold for all 36 years old and, as a rule of thumb, patients who are older are usually proposed adapted psychotherapeutic support. Thought processes cannot be changed that easily.

3. François

François, aged six and with a brother who is three years older, arrives at the autism resource centre for an opinion concerning his diagnosis. Pregnancy and birth were without complications and he was breastfed for four months, the first stages of development were then normal, he could sit at seven months, walk at fourteen months and toilet training (day and night) was acquired at thirty months. However, when he is around two years old, François's parents started to worry because he was not speaking and had a peculiar way of looking at objects and people, never fully engaging in an interaction with them. Food had to be mashed, François refused to eat pieces. Language did appear six months later but it remained limited to a few words and stereotypical sentences. The parents took François in for a consultation when he was three and a half. Patient care was put in place, starting with weekly speech therapy, psychomotor therapy, and psychotherapy. The child psychiatrist finally concluded that he had 'severe' autism and proposed that patient care be continued at a day hospital, for four half-days a week during two years. The hospital team further proposed to strengthen the care and to take François in full-time, which his parents refused as they still wished that he attended school at least part-time. The divergence in opinion with the child psychiatrist became such that the parents decided to stop the care and organised speech and psychomotor therapy with practitioners based in the city.

François's medical records are particular because he suffered from AV nodal re-entrant tachycardia at two years old, prior to supraventricular tachycardial episodes. During a tachycardial episode, he had a convulsive fit. He was prescribed Cordarone®, which prevented the episodes and convulsive fits. He also underwent an adenoidectomy at eighteen months due to recurring ear aches.

During his first consultation, I observed a child who made sparse use of language. Exchanges were rare, only of his initiative, and concerned just simple requests for a toy or for something to eat or drink. He aligned toy animals and did not allow his brother to take one. His movements were stereotyped when he is excited or frustrated. Most of the time, he smiled and gave the impression of being rather impermeable to others' emotions. At night, when it was time for sleep, François easily accepted to go bed but, once his bedroom door was closed, he would get up and play silently for many hours before falling asleep. I proposed to his parents that they try melatonin (close to 60% of autistic children have trouble falling asleep, which is linked to a lack of circadian secretion of melatonin). For François, taking 1 mg of melatonin when going to bed allowed him to fall asleep in half an hour (it is a treatment that induces sleep without prolonged sedative effects).

The evaluation conducted at the autism resource centre confirmed the autism diagnosis. François was hypersensitive to sounds and touch. His spontaneous activities were not properly performed but, when we adapted him to the situations, he performed at a level equal to that of other children his own age. For example, during a three-dimensional constructive praxis test, François completed the first two tasks without adaptation being required, whilst the more complex third task was completed once we provided him the pieces one by one to limit the stimuli that reached him. The speech therapy evaluation concluded that there had been a delay in language establishing itself with regards to all speech components (voice, articulation, vocabulary, syntax, and pragmatics). Often, François gave the impression that he was speaking to himself, but sometimes he paradoxically asked small questions to his discussion partner ('What are you doing?, 'Why are you doing that?'). He asked these questions when he was surprised by an adult's behaviour and listened to the reply, sometimes signifying his approval or disapproval to the answer. The key parts of the evaluation were dedicated to repetitive tasks where he explored objects. He had a lot of difficulty with engaging in the building of a game scenario from the moment that he tries to put in place the necessary basic oppositions (inside-out, opened-closed…).

François was six years old when this evaluation was made and his parents agreed to participate in the trial the next year, when he was seven. If we want to show that bumetanide is beneficial for treating autism, it is important that these children do not take any other treatment during the trial period (if they did, how would we know which treatment is the successful one?). But sleep deprivation tires both the child and the parents – it is often the symptom that is coped with least easily, causing progressive exhaustion and its parade of associated difficulties (annoyance, animosity, anxiety, and sometimes mood swings). Indeed, it is so acute that we do not want to ask the parents to return to those times just to undertake a trial. Moreover, a lot of publications that investigate melatonin and autism show that its effect is limited to inducing sleep. So we decided not to stop the melatonin treatment while we underwent the trial. At the end of the trial, the parents requested that we continue the bumetanide prescription. From the first days of the treatment, they reported back saying that François has stopped circling the table (which he could do many times a day, sometimes for a long time) but that it was with time that changes become truly visible. François was schooled in a regular classroom, he repeated year 2 (1st grade) and therefore he was only in year 4 (3rd grade) and followed by a paraprofessional. He continued speech therapy, but psychomotor re-education stopped and writing difficulties led to an occupational therapist being enlisted. After 16 months of treatment, a speech therapy review underlined that he was slow to develop speech and language, encountering difficulties when it came to syntactic construction (his aptitudes matched those of a child in year 3 (2nd grade)). He could read small sentences and write using capital letters. The speech therapist concluded by stating that François was cooperative, diligent, and sought to do well. His behaviour exhibited clear progress, he accepted constraints and the timer need only be used for the more boring exercises (writing). His ability to visualise the various activities of each session was not systematically required anymore. As to his schooling, François enjoys attending for the first time this year and wants to do the same work as the others. The teacher notes that he is more adaptable and communicates with her. Up until now all communication took place via the paraprofessional. He approaches other students, looks at what they are doing, speaks to them, especially during recess, and he accepts without difficulty changes in his desk neighbour.

His parents also note that François now complains when he hurts himself but these complaints are not excessive – it is as if his perception of pain has been normalised. His behavioural problems that are due to neuro-sensorial annoyance are less frequent. Indeed, some noises and smells used to trigger tantrums in François. He would put his hands on his ears and exhibit motor stereotypies and complete relational incapacity. These difficulties would end as quickly as they had appeared once the irritating stimulus stops. His family would previously be careful to avoid such stimuli but this is not the case today – sometimes he even seeks them. To clean the car, the family goes to the nearby garage that has an automatic car wash. His brother would like to stay in the car, looking at the hubbub of the cleaning rolls. François would always move away; the sound would be unbearable for him. Now, he remains with his brother in the car, laughing heartily at the experience.

4. Hector

Hector has a twin sister, Lola. They were both term babies, born in autumn 1997 following a calm pregnancy. When Hector was nursing, he was difficult to feed as he did not suckle properly. He was nevertheless an energetic and lively baby. His parents located a break in his development at around four months, when he suddenly became apathetic, had trouble sleeping, and developed congenital torticollis. At seven months, his slowdown was such that they consult the CAMPS autism resource centre. During the consultation, Hector locked eyes well, smiled, cooed, and gurgled. We noted, however, that he was reacting little to sound (though his hearing evaluation was normal) and that he was hypotonic and already exhibiting psychomotor slowdown. The paraclinical evaluation (neuro-paediatric, genetic, ophthalmologic, and ORL) was completely normal.

During a consultation at twenty-eight months, the doctor noted that his communication was very poor. Hector only made monosyllabic sounds without communicating anything of substance. There was a dearth of symbolic games and little social interactions, without proto-declarative pointing or joint attention. He did not maintain eye contact and did not seem to get pleasure from cuddling. Sometimes he would laugh wholeheartedly but for no obvious reason. He did not yet walk and refused food when in pieces. At thirty months, a diagnostic evaluation was made at the autism resource centre and it concluded that he has severe autism with developmental delay. His developmental stage was deemed at eleven months for posture, seven months for speech, five months for hand-eye coordination, and four months for socialisation. Hector was then welcomed into a day hospital, where the patient care was first for two hours per week but then increased over time. At six years old he was taken into care at a medical-educational treatment centre.

Hector was eleven years old when he started taking bumetanide. At the time he had difficulty walking. He could not climb stairs so his mother carried him to reach my office. I rarely locked eyes with him – he spent most of his time immersed in solitary activities that are very repetitive and poor in stimulation, sometimes shaking the object in front of his face and throwing away the toys we give him. His sister was the only one able to have a few exchanges with him and, even if they were short, they encouraged us to pursue our efforts. He shouted out often, was impulsive, irritable, and agitated. It was difficult to read his facial emotions; he spent a lot of time looking into space with a frozen expression. His developmental stage was deemed to be at eleven months. After three months of treatment, we noted a small improvement. His behaviour and attitudes remain particular but it is easier to get him to emerge from them. Then, as months went by, Hector started to climb up and down stairs with help, he gave us toys and enjoyed games involving exchange. He continued to shout and cry out, but did so less and less. In particular, his verbal output was enriched by monosyllabic words that were uttered at well-timed moments. He could remain seated calmly during meals. Even if his progress remained very slow, the change contrasted drastically with the situation pre-treatment when he had gained just a few months of development in eight years.

From that point on, hundreds of children started getting treated with bumetanide, sometimes for up to three years and often with impressive effects. This suggests that continued treatment can very much improve the evolution of the disorder. Of course, we had to develop extra trials in parallel to test the medicine on a larger scale and to then obtain the authorisation for placing it on the market (as we will see later). In between, however, new possibilities allowed us to expand our understanding of the diuretic's effects and its action in other areas used to measure autism.

IV

AUTISM'S GAZE, COMMUNICATION DIFFICULTIES, AND BUMETANIDE

1. Brain imaging to the rescue: what if certain brain circuits were not – or too much activated? Look me in the eyes!

One of the things that is striking when meeting an autistic person is that it is difficult to maintain eye contact (Robison, 2008). What causes this gaze avoidance and what is it, really?

About a decade ago, Ami Klin, a researcher at Yale, had the brilliant idea of using an eye-tracker whilst showing scenes of Mike Nichols' film of Edward Albee's play, 'Who's afraid of Virginia Woolf?'. Its scenario follows fast-moving interactions between two university couples in an American campus house. There are only social interactions, which is something particularly difficult for autistic people to deal with. The eye-tracker allows one to know exactly where people are looking thanks to a system of infrared captors, and allows us to see what an autistic person focuses on as they are looking at these images, and to better understand why it may be difficult for them to understand these social interactions: A neurotypical person has a tendency to go from one face to the next in order to understand the actions and intentions of the protagonists. An autistic person, who may have a completely normal level of intelligence, will focus on the scene's details and not on the characters, and even less on their faces or their eyes. It is therefore not surprising that they cannot grasp all the non-verbal interactions and, in particular, the gazes people give each other.

This technique can now be used in routine laboratory research coupled with a system that measures the responses and reaction times. The eye-tracker is a tool that at first sight seems like a simple computer screen. Its bottom part has infrared cameras that allow it to capture the position and the size of each pupil with great temporal and spatial precision (the system takes 120 measurements per second, and can detect a difference of gaze of 11mm on a screen at a distance of 65cm). To carry out an experiment with the eye-tracker, one just needs to sit in front of the screen and to calibrate it (which takes only a few seconds). Then, participants look at the images that appear on the screen. These will depend on what the researcher wants to examine. This research method is used for people of all ages, even babies, who can sit on the lap of the person accompanying them. Recently, marketing companies have also started to use this technology to monitor perception when people view their advertising pages or websites. Thanks to this system, we can precisely know (down to a few degrees of angle) where a person spontaneously looks when they first see an image, what they look at and for how long, and what interests them or not. This is a windfall for researchers as, for the first time, they can find out exactly what visual exploratory behaviour is taking place in their subject. This allows them to truly 'walk in their shoes' or, better still, 'see through their eyes' (Guillon, Hadjikhani, Baduel, & Roge, 2014).

We quickly learned that this technique would be of great use to us to finally understand how autistic people view the world and faces in particular. If we show an autistic person some faces expressing different emotions and ask them to categorise them, they are slower and make more mistakes than the 'control' group members of the same age and intelligence. We also note that they spend less time than neurotypical people when looking into the eye area of faces. Why do they avoid gazes? For the moment, we have no answer to this question. When we ask an autistic person why they do not make eye contact, we often get the reply that it is 'too much', 'too intense', 'as if it burns', and that it requires too much effort. But why?

One of the possible reasons is that the brain's structure in charge of detecting relevant elements in our surroundings, the amygdala, is activated too much in autistic people. This would lead them to actively look away when they have to meet another's gaze in the same way that we look away when faced with a horrific scene or a dramatic accident. Gaze avoidance may stem from an abnormally excitable brain at birth. Here is our hypothesis (which so far is only a hypothesis, but that with time will be either proven right or rejected):

The subcortical face processing pathway, that consists of the superior colliculus, the pulvinar nucleus of the thalamus, and the amygdala, is a fast 'low-tech' processing pathway that is already functional at birth. Newborns preferentially orient towards faces, as demonstrated by Mark H. Johnson in the 1990s (Johnson, Dziurawiec, Ellis, & Morton, 1991). In fact, this seems to happen even before birth, as a recent study showed that human foetuses have a preference for 'protofaces' (stimuli that consist of three dots that look like two eyes and a mouth) (Reid et al., 2017). This system allows newborns to be extraordinarily sensitive to faces, to orient towards them, and to get the necessary exposure needed for the normal the maturation of the visual areas that will become the cortical face processing system, and allow the development of what we can call "the social brain" (Brothers, 1990).

Now, imagine that at birth there is too much excitatory input, because there is too much chloride in the cells, and that GABA cannot perform its inhibitory function. Newborn see, most of their time awake, faces of caregivers. This activates the subcortical system, but in the case of autism, it activates it too much, because the brain is hyperexcitable, and according to the Hebbian rules, "what fires together wires together", therefore the entire system, including the amygdala, becomes hyperconnected. The subcortical system is also sensitive to eyes, and to eye contact in particular. Eye contact is a crucial way to communicate without using words, and it is also very important for the development of language, as it provides deictic information, linking objects with words, for example. An abnormally connected subcortical system would result in the fact that the amygdala would become hypersensitive to eye contact. At that point, eye contact would be experienced as stressful, or threatening, and therefore avoided. Turning away from faces and from direct gaze would result in a reduction of exposure to other people's eyes and faces, which would then in turn result in an abnormal experience and therefore an abnormal development of the social brain, including areas of the mirror system. In addition, it would result in difficulties in language acquisition, and therefore affect both social and communication abilities. Our research indicates that there is indeed some evidence that this hypothesis may be right (see below, in the last chapter entitled six years later), and that rather than being indifferent to others, people with autism may actually be oversensitive to others, and that avoiding eye contact is a way to cope with this feeling of being overwhelmed.

Besides not controlling for gaze, many studies that look at face perception in autism have another problem, as most of the time they show face stimuli that have exaggerated facial expression, which are almost never encountered in everyday life (with an interesting exception: when a caregiver talks to a baby, all facial expressions seem to be generated in a very much amplified way, as if to teach the child the basics of the way emotions are expressed). What happens with faces that look more like what we encounter in our daily life? To address this question, we created faces with more subtle emotions by using a software that allows to morph between, for example, a neutral and a fearful face, and we presented faces with only 40% of the full emotional intensity, with a cross in the eye region to ensure that participants would look in the eyes. Unexpectedly (or maybe not really, given our previous observations), we observed that individuals with autism were in fact hypersensitive to the faces that were expressing fear at 40% intensity compared with controls, as evidenced by more amygdala activation in the autism group (Lassalle et al., 2017). This is more evidence that the threat detection system may be oversensitive in autism, and that gaze avoidance results as a coping mechanism to reduce stress.

This has important implications, in terms of therapy: a lot of cognitive behavioral approaches (e.g. Applied Behavioral Analysis, ABA) are based on the positive reinforcement of appropriate behavior, and eye contact is considered to be an appropriate behavior. For example, when playing together with their child, parents are told that they should suddenly stop the fun game and request that their child will look them in the eyes in exchange for a treat, that will be given to them only give once eye contact is established. This may be a good approach if children are indifferent to eye contact. But if they are indeed oversensitive, which seems to be the case in at least a good proportion of them (as evidenced by research showing increased pupil size, increased heart rate, increased galvanic skin response, and increased amygdala activation during eye contact), then forcing children with autism to establish eye contact may not be the appropriate way to help them, and maybe another approach may be less stressful and more efficient. This approach would consist in a program that would desensitize, or habituate them to make eye contact, creating less anxiety for the child, and help them slowly, at their pace, confront eye gaze, in a way similar to which a medical student slowly habituates to seeing blood and viscera during the course of medical school.

In addition to showing that autistic individuals are oversensitive to faces subtly expressing fear (Lassalle et al., 2017), we recently demonstrated that their amygdala gets overactivated when they are constrained to look in the eyes (N. Hadjikhani et al., 2017).

We can use eye-tracking techniques to follow the autistic person's gaze and determine whether they are looking into another's eyes. We can use a task where they must recognise ambiguous emotions to determine the accurateness of their replies and their reaction time. In parallel, we can use imagery techniques to determine whether the brain regions that are activated by emotionally expressive faces shake up the brain networks similarly or differently than in neurotypical people. We then at once better understand how the brain's functioning and the causes of neurological disorders are linked and whether intervention to create some order is possible. New techniques of brain imagery and new measures with which to assess behaviour allow us to better comprehend the anatomic and functional foundations of the difference between the brains of autistic people and those of people with a 'typical' development. They will also soon allow us to rigorously and objectively follow the impact of treatments not just on behaviour but on the brain's structure too.

With the eye-tracking technology, we can also measure pupil size, which is an important marker of inner state, including levels of stress. We have performed experiments that have shown that when we ask individuals with autism to look in the eyes, their pupil becomes much wider than that of typical controls, indicating higher level of arousal/stress. In addition to that, we have been looking at an interesting phenomenon called pupillary contagion, which consists of an involuntary change on one's pupil size to adapt to that of another person. This phenomenon seems to be important in the transfer of affective and arousal levels between people. We recently examined whether this contagion would be present in autism. To do so, we created stimuli that were happy and sad faces of avatar females and manipulated the size of the pupil, and presented each face twice, once with a small, and once with a large pupil. Participants were not made aware of this, and were simply asked to attentively look at the faces, which were shown in random order. To our surprise, we found a robust pupil mimicry effect both in the participants with autism and in the controls, and this effect did not differ between groups. In fact, if anything, it happened faster in those with autism, showing that even if they look less at the eyes, individuals with autism respond strongly to the level of arousal transmitted from others, and that they may in fact be oversensitive to other people's emotion, even at an unconscious level, since pupillary mimicry is an involuntary phenomenon (Galazka et al., 2018).

We conclude from all these studies that eye-contact avoidance in people with ASD is in fact a way to reduce the stress perceived, a strategy that is coming at some costs, of course, not only because 'typical' people tend to distrust those who do not look them in the eyes, or think they are not interested – but also because we learn so much about the state of mind of others by the information that is displayed by the eyes that those with ASD who avoid looking there not only have difficulties interpreting emotions, but also less training in learning about them.

Not looking in the eyes has indeed important repercussions. It is very difficult for an autistic person to read the emotions expressed on a face, especially when they are not exaggerated – as is usually the case in daily life. There are many reasons for this.

The first is the most obvious. The consequence of gaze aversion is that autistic people become less able than neurotypical people to read the subtle signals constantly emitted by faces (both with regards to their intensity and their duration) because they are looking at people less. The second is rooted in the normal circuitry that is usually involved in the reading of emotions. It seems that we do not understand an emotion intimately unless we reproduce it ourselves, even without realising it. This was demonstrated in the 1980s by a Swedish researcher, Ulf Dimberg (Dimberg, 1982). He made his 'normal' subjects look at faces that expressed different emotions while simultaneously recording the contraction in their facial muscles that are used to smile or wrinkle our brow. He noted that when we see a face that smiles, we automatically (in just 200 milliseconds) contract our own smile muscles, the zygomatics. On the other hand, when we perceive an angry face, we contract our corrugator, the muscle that make us wrinkle our brow. All this happens without us realising it. We can follow this even further: the same phenomenon happens even if the emotional face is presented subliminally, without time for us to realise that we have seen it. Finally, his group demonstrated that the amount of muscular activation of the face is correlated with the subject's empathy, the degree of which is measured using questionnaires. (Funnily, injecting Botox® paralyses the little muscles of the face that allow emotions to express themselves, which means that a person who had a Botox® injection is less able to understand emotion in others…) When we carry out the same experiment in autistic people by showing them faces expressing emotions, nothing happens: they do not exhibit this automatic mimicry. In other words, quasi-automatic mimicry reaction to the perception of emotion does not work well in autistic people.

In the 2000s, researchers decided to use brain imaging to look at what goes on in the brain of an autistic person when they are shown faces. To do that, the researchers showed pairs of faces or objects to autistic people and to neurotypical controls, who had to say whether the images were similar or different. The researchers observed the activation in the area of the brain that is dedicated to identifying faces, the fusiform face area (FFA) only in controls. The authors promptly declared that autistic people behaved with others as if they were objects because they could not differentiate between faces and objects, as they simply did not have a functioning FFA. It was a simple explanation, easy to understand, satisfactory. Except that… Were the autistic people actually looking at the faces that were presented? If neurotypical people spontaneously carry out the task of matching between faces by looking in particular at the eye region, autistic people may be using completely different techniques. Our team showed, sometime later, that if we constrained autistic people to look in the eye region by placing a cross in the middle of the face, the FFA would get activated in them just as in the control group (N. Hadjikhani et al., 2004). It was then established that, in fact, the activation in this region is directly linked to the time spent looking in the eye area and that this is true in both autistic (Dalton et al., 2005) and neurotypical people (Morris, Pelphrey, & McCarthy, 2007). And as mentioned above, we also showed that constraining autistic people to look in the eyes resulted in abnormal amygdala elevation (N. Hadjikhani et al., 2017).

There are, however, other differences in brain activation in response to the perception of faces. Perceiving a face is the product of a collaboration within a whole network of brain areas, which are not only linked to face perception but also to perceiving emotions and intentions. As mentioned above, newborns preferentially orient towards faces, thanks to the subcortical system. But it gets even more impressive, as shown by Andrew N. Meltzoff in the 1970s: when we stick our tongue out at a newborn, they will stick out theirs in imitation, even if they have been born for just a few minutes. What does this mean? What is so impressive about that? Let us pause for a while to understand what needs to happen for such a phenomenon to be possible. The baby has just been born. She has been seeing for a few minutes and has never seen a face. She finds herself face to face with someone who is sticking their tongue out and she is capable, spontaneously and instinctively, to imitate. She 'knows' that what she sees is a face, a mouth, and a tongue, and that she herself has a face, a mouth, and a tongue. She observes that the person is using their muscles to stick their tongue out and she 'knows' which muscles she must herself use to produce the same action. All this is in fact very complex. But it is also innate. We arrive in this world with a brain that allows us to imitate, thanks to particularly intriguing neurons called 'mirror neurons'.

2. Mirror neurons: a basis for social and emotional understanding?

Mirror neurons were discovered in monkeys at the end of the 1990s by Giacomo Rizzolatti's team in Parma (Rizzolatti & Fabbri-Destro, 2010). The researchers were recording what they thought were purely motor neurons, those involved in triggering action. They realised by chance that these neurons were actually activated when the monkey was observing someone doing the same action as that which the neurons would be specialised for, without that monkey doing anything itself. Everything was happening as if the neurons were anticipating the nature of the movements that the person in front of the monkey was doing and, in a way, was mimicking them. The team baptised these neurons 'mirror neurons', an apt name indeed.

What do these mirror neurons do? What is their purpose? By being active when we do something and when we see the same action effected by another, they allow us to put ourselves in the other's place, to adopt their point of view. Thanks to them, we can both imitate and know the intentions and emotions of others better, as we saw above with the automatic imitations of a smile or anger. These neurons are therefore good candidates for the formation of social and emotional understanding with others, allowing us to do what another is doing or feel what another is enduring…

When we show a smiling face to a neurotypical person, a group of brain areas activate one by one in a few hundreds of milliseconds. In a way, we can observe and dissect the brain structures that take part in these actions thanks to magnetoencephalography, which allows us to precisely record the tiny magnetic currents generated by neurons' electric discharges down to the millisecond. This technique allows us to create short movies depicting the activation of different parts of the brain in real time and to highlight the complexity of the situation and the number of actors that are present during the hundreds of milliseconds that follow seeing a face, for example. Thanks to functional MRIs, which collect images over two or three seconds, we can precisely determine the location of the main actors in recognition and try to answer the following question: what does my brain do when I identify the meaning of a face? The answer: a collection of regions that years of experimental research have uncovered and characterised as involved in this identification process' many facets. Perceiving and interpreting a smiling face is not simple. I must at the same time translate the physical properties of this image and compare it to the hundred others I have learned to identify in their context and texture throughout my life, as well as the memories I have of these shapes. The brain is memory, as biologists often declare. For this reconstruction, I need to group all this information together and identify which will without doubt allow full and complete identification of the face. Expressive faces trigger areas of the brain involved in the identification of faces, such as the FFA as well as areas engaged in the treatment of emotions, like the amygdala. They also trigger areas involved in the interpretation of biological movements, such as the superior temporal sulcus, or other areas involved in facial mimicry, such as the somatomotor cortex for the face, and the areas relevant to the mirror mechanisms, the inferior frontal gyrus and the inferior parietal cortex. It is the activation of this collective of structures and neural networks that allow us to identify the content of these images with certainty.

What do we observe in autistic people? As we have seen above, the areas of the brain that identify faces activate normally. Contrary to neurotypical people, however, those with autism do not spontaneously activate the superior temporal sulcus, the right amygdala, or the mirror and somatomotor areas for mimicry (N. Hadjikhani et al., 2009; N. Hadjikhani, Joseph, Snyder, & Tager-Flusberg, 2007). Their 'social brain' is not activated at all. It is as if the autistic person cannot give texture to the image, as if it does not 'speak' to him and does not evoke a memory because the corresponding file is not in his library of images.

What else do we observe that could hint to a dysfunctional mirror mechanism in autism? Contagious yawning, a phenomenon we all know well, is a good example. All mammals yawn, even *in utero*, but few are prone to contagious yawning. It develops in children between one and two years of age and is easily triggered when seeing others yawn. Researchers have observed that people with high levels of empathy are more susceptible to contagious yawning. This contagion is shown to be much less present in autistic children and adults than in neurotypical people (Helt, Eigsti, Snyder, & Fein, 2010).

This brings us to empathy. What is empathy? By definition, it is the ability to share and 'understand' the emotions of others by feeling them ourselves. One of autism's characteristics is the *impression of a lack of empathy* towards others, which is exhibited very early on – it can be observed already from two years of age. Is it really a lack of empathy or is it rather the absence of empathetic behaviour? What is the role of the mirror mechanisms? When we perceive others' emotions, we use the same parts of our brain that we would use if we were to feel them ourselves. We have been able to show that, for example, following the injury of a part of the brain called the insula, which is important for feeling internal sensations and experiencing disgust, patients become suddenly unable to perceive when a person in front of them winces in disgust but they remain perfectly able to recognise a smile or anger. Other researchers have also shown that if a part of the brain that receives and triggers information from the face's muscles is damaged following a stroke, they cannot perform facial mimicry and become unable to recognise any emotion. We also know that to adopt a facial expression generates activity in the autonomous system specific to that expression. Edgar Allan Poe illustrates this well in his short story, 'The Purloined Letter': 'When I wish to find out how wise, or how stupid, or how good, or how wicked is any one, or what are his thoughts at the moment, I fashion the expression of my face, as accurately as possible, in accordance with the expression of his, and then wait to see what thoughts or sentiments arise in my mind or heart, as if to match or correspond with the expression.'

It therefore seems that mirror mechanisms play a key role in the perception of emotions. By activating these regions of the brain, I mime the actions of my correspondent and, in a way, relive them. I am therefore able to feel the benefits and harm. Not being able to perceive the emotions in oneself makes it difficult to then appreciate its nuances. Mirroring deficiencies in autistic people impede them to feel emotions in others.

Nothing is simple, however. If autistic people have a hard time reading certain emotions, that does not make them indifferent to others. In fact, it seems that the opposite is often true. We conducted an experiment during which we showed faces expressing pain to people with autism and to a control group (N. Hadjikhani et al., 2014). We believed that we would demonstrate that the face expressing pain would not trigger any more activation in the brain of autistic people than showing a neutral face. So we were very surprised when we realised that the two groups had the same amount of activation in the areas of the brain that are involved in the perception of pain, thus displaying 'affective' or 'emotional' empathy. But other regions of the brain that are important for 'cognitive' empathy or theory of mind, such as the medial prefrontal cortex, were only activated in the control group. Additionally, what differentiated the two groups was more activation in autistic people of an area involved in reappraisal (the dorsolateral prefrontal cortex), which is the same area that is activated in doctors when they observe a patient who is suffering. It seems that an autistic person who sees a distressed person also experiences that distress but is unable to 'mentalise' it as neurotypical people do. If autistic people seem to be distancing themselves and seem not care about others, it is in fact because they are overwhelmed by their emotions and therefore trying to protect themselves by withdrawing.

However, when we compared the results of this study with those from another study where we presented stimuli showing hands or feet that were being stabbed, or pricked with a syringe, etc, surely eliciting pain in the (unseen) owner of these hands and feet, we saw that those with autism in fact had less activation than the controls in the areas of the mirror system, showing that it was for them more difficult to embody the perceived pain when there was not clear facial expression of pain being shown (in which case they had the same if not more activation than the controls) (Lassalle et al., 2018).

So the lack of empathy in autistic people is a more complex problem than we would have thought of at the start. And maybe, it is because the word empathy itself also poses a problem, because it means so many different things, and covers so many different concepts. There are in fact two major types of empathy, that we can call *cognitive* and *affective*. *Cognitive empathy* is the capacity that we have to take someone else's perspective, to "put ourselves in their shoes". It is a rather complicated thing to do, as it requests to override our point of view, our knowledge, and to see the world from another perspective. Some also call it Theory of Mind. Being able to infer other people's mental states is important in order to understand and predict their behaviour. We know which brain areas are mostly involved in cognitive empathy (the medial prefrontal cortex, the right temporo-parietal junction and superior temporal sulcus – that is, mirror mechanisms together with areas involved in mental state attribution). Individuals with autism struggle with cognitive empathy, and sometimes may have a very difficult time seeing things from someone else's perspective.

Affective empathy makes you share the feelings of the person you interact with or observe. It is the process by which you wince in pain when you hear the story of someone getting their fingers snapped in a doorway, or when you perceive the face of someone in extreme pain. Brain imaging studies have demonstrated that all the areas that are activated when you experience pain (also known as the pain matrix) are also activated to a certain extent when you observe or think about these painful events. This capacity to "suffer with" is not affected in individuals with autism, who are as sensitive as we are to the perception of people expressing pain. In fact, they may be even more sensitive than we are, as it is difficult for them to take distance, and not feel overwhelmed by witnessing pain – and the only reason they may not display the caring, consoling behaviour that one would expect, is that they experience personal distress and need to take distance in order to not feel overwhelmed.

As long as we use one single word to express two very different realities, we will have difficulties understanding each other and communicating. We will be confused when we read things as opposite as "empathy is a bad thing that precludes rational thinking" (Paul Bloom), or discover that there is a program to improve our empathy in 5, 6, or 7 steps. Clearly stated concepts are extremely important if we want to stop spreading confusion by talking about very different notions using one term. We need to recognize that autism is not a disorder of empathy, but rather a condition in which cognitive empathy is reduced, but affective empathy is heightened, which can lead to very stressful situations in their daily life.

We have said above that these mirror mechanisms are important for learning by imitation, something that is deficient in autistic people, and for understanding the actions and emotions of others. These areas do not seem to function normally in autistic people but what role do they play exactly? And why do they seem to not function normally? Scientists have ascertained an anatomical and functional anomaly in these regions by looking at the relevant brain areas in autistic people. Are these differences the cause or the consequence of autism? It is also both interesting and important to note that these mirror mechanisms are normally employed when perceiving certain movements and stimuli that hail back to the most ancient ontological survival mechanisms, of which pain is one. So it is not the mirror mechanisms themselves that seem affected by autism but rather the fact that they are not triggered spontaneously during the perception of social stimuli.

3. Pilot studies on the effects of bumetanide

The observations made by Dr Éric Lemonnier and the parents of children treated with bumetanide showed that there was an improvement in the symptoms but that we now needed to quantify these effects by using techniques that would allow us to determine what objective modifications were produced by this improvement. We therefore threw ourselves into this big project, which was possible only thanks to the incredible willingness of the participants and their parents, and the collaboration of motivated and enthusiastic teams.

Everything started with Dr Lemonnier contacting a number of his patients to ask whether a trip to Switzerland, including a little bonus brain MRI followed by an eye-tracking exam, might tempt them. Many families rose to the challenge of travelling from Brest and staying a few days in Lausanne to undergo the tests. Upon their return to Brest, the patients underwent the bumetanide treatment under the watchful eye of Dr Lemonnier and, ten months later, they returned to Switzerland. Taken under the wing of Nouchine Hadjikhani and her team in Lausanne, the teens visibly enjoyed the experience – they asked if they could return soon!

For each visit, the participants underwent a series of psychological tests, during which they had to fill in questionnaires and undergo eye-tracking and functional MRI examinations. The results greatly surpassed our expectations (N. Hadjikhani et al., 2015). We observed that, after the bumetanide treatment, our participants' performance saw a change not just in the terms of behaviour but also in imagery. One of the tests was an emotion matching task. On the left side, a face was presented that expresses emotions (joy, fear, anger) of an intensity set at 40%, whilst, on the right, another person's face either expresses one of three emotions at 100% or a neutral one. Each image has a number and the task is to push on the number that corresponds to the low-intensity (40%) emotion expressed on the left. We never tell the participant whether the answer they select is right or wrong, so that the right answer remains a mystery to them for the rest of the exercise. To ensure that the classification concept is well understood, we also show images of animals, musical instruments, clothes and fruits, which have to be matched by category.

What did we notice after the treatment? It was apparent that the participants not only became faster for the emotion assessment task, but they also performed with fewer mistakes than before the treatment. In fact, their performance arrived close to that of the neurotypical control participants. The benefit of this measure, compared to a standard behaviour questionnaire or observation by a psychologist or a parent, is that it is objective. It measures how long it takes to push the button and how often the participants are deceived by the task. From this, we produced statistics that show a significant improvement. And the brain, in all this? Were we able to measure the effect of the treatment? Well yes, and we will illustrate the results obtained with one of the imaging tests. In this experiment, the participants watched short films lasting a few seconds, with faces that went from neutral to expressive. The expressions, as before, were of joy, fear, or anger. The neutral one sometimes changed in orientation so that a sense of movement was created. As we know that brain activity changes when one concentrates on emotion during the perception of faces, we gave a task that would not influence the results but that would ensure that the participants were sensitive to stimuli presented to them: a cross, which appears levelled to the eyes, changes from red to blue every now and then, and participants had to press a button to signal when they observed a blue cross.

When analysing the results, we compared the difference in brain activation between each of the emotions and the neutral condition, to expose areas of the brain that are involved in the perception of emotions. We saw that there was practically no difference in activation before the bumetanide treatment between a face that expresses an emotion and a neutral face: the tested emotions appear to be badly decoded by the brain. By contrast, in the second imaging session that took place after the patients had taken the bumetanide for several months, we observed that all of a sudden, the zones in the brain that are important for social communication, including the upper temporal gyrus, were now activated during emotional perception (N. Hadjikhani et al., 2015).

We also looked at the effect of treatment on amygdala activation, and on eye contact (Nouchine Hadjikhani et al., 2018). As mentioned above, we had shown that constraining autistic individuals to look in the eyes provoked abnormal amygdala activation (N. Hadjikhani et al., 2017) – the question now was: what happens after 10 months of bumetanide treatment? And the response was beyond our expectations: Not only did bumetanide treatment for 10 months normalize activation in the amygdala when individuals with ASD were 'forced' to look in the eyes, but it also increased the time that they would spontaneously spend looking in the eyes when looking at faces, as measured by an eye-tracking system. This demonstrates that bumetanide treatment may improve social processing in autism, even in young adults, and not only in children.

Of course, one could say that this effect can be attributed to the passing of time and that the participants were more comfortable the second time. To ensure that this was not the case, we also tested two young citizens of Brest who had not taken the bumetanide but who had experienced the same protocol as the rest of the team. At home, no notable change occurred between the first and second time, their brain continued to respond indifferently when comparing emotive and neutral faces. These pilot, proof-of-concept experiments concerned only a small group of participants. Larger-scale studies will have to be done, along with a double-blind study, to confirm these initial results. But they are nonetheless extremely encouraging and we look forward to continuing this great adventure.

In conclusion, these insights converge and strengthen the possibility of using a diuretic as a treatment for autism. At this stage, we have no idea if the premise of this investigation is valid: is the concentration of intracellular chloride high? Indeed, the fact that the diuretic is beneficial could be explained, for example, by remote actions on the periphery. Naturally, measuring the chloride concentrations in the human brain has to be excluded, at least with autism, because we do not have the surgical appliances with which one could make these measurements. This is not the case in childhood epilepsies or adults who can have defective areas surgically removed, as with the formation of a double cortex (which we looked at previously). Work carried out on these cases effectively exhibits high concentrations of chloride and GABA's excitatory action. We therefore turned to mice to study the links between GABA actions, autism, and birth with the assumption that the GABA developmental shift might be altered in relation with the pathogenesis of autism.

4. Studies on 'autistic' mice confirm our hypothesis and the role of childbirth

Admittedly, the jump from epilepsies to autism is not straightforward! Experimental observations suggest that the Excitation/Inhibition balance is tilted in favour of excitation in autism and epilepsies and 30% of children with autism have also seizures. In animal models of autism there is a reduction of the threshold to generate seizures. Yet, things are not as simple as not all epileptic children have autistic features and conversely not all children with autism have epileptic events. Here also animal models are instrumental to determine underlying mechanisms. There are many rodent models thought to reproduce some features of autism and used to determine effects of drugs and treatments. Most of them rely on producing mice usually with genetic mutations that are also observed in humans. However, extensive clinical observations in humans first obtained several decades ago suggest that maternal use of an antiepileptic agent called Sodium Valproate (Depakine) leads to autism spectrum disorders in off spring. Similar apparent "autistic" features are observed in rodent treated during gestation with this drug. We adopted this model as it is quite reliable and reproducible. We also used the Fragile X genetic syndrome that is associated with autistic like behavioural features. In spite of their obvious differences, they are quite complementary stressing the similarities with some cardinal features of autism and most notably social interactions. Pups with either pathological condition emit characteristic vocalisations when they are separated from their mothers and avoid novelty. Also, when facing a choice between a familiar and an unfamiliar one, they will prefer the former whereas mice with autism prefer exploring novel environment and mouse they have not met previously. Admittedly, this falls short of the complications of autism in infants, but electrical and morphological observations suggest common structural basis. Therefore, in spite of the major difference between different animal species, these models can provide useful information in spite of their limitations in particular on possible underlying mechanisms and actions of candidate treatments. They are indispensable to determine whether indeed chloride levels are impacted in autism and restored by bumetanide.

This ensemble of data is compatible with the initial hypothesis that using a diuretic can correct high concentrations of chloride but this remains to be demonstrated. Indeed, bumetanide may exert its effects through other actions, whether peripheral or central. Moreover, as this molecule has a short lifespan *in vivo* (it degrades quickly and penetrates badly through the brain) hypotheses other than ours cannot be excluded. Consequently, it must be directly demonstrated that neurons have high concentrations of chloride in autism and that bumetanide can reduce it. To reach this conclusion, there is one option: the use of autistic animals as a model, given that chloride concentrations cannot be measured in human tissue. Although the disease is only very partially mimicked by these model animals, there are enough similar properties on a morphological, biochemical, and physiological basis for data to confirm or contradict the hypothesis. Thus, an epileptic pregnant rat given an antiepileptic drug (valproate) during pregnancy can give birth to 'autistic' offspring. This is observed in humans too. In the same way, the mutation of certain genes or invalidation of a part of the X chromosome (the X-fragile) leads, in both humans and rats, to autistic syndromes. We can therefore use rodents to determine the excitatory actions of GABA and whether chloride levels are high.

As a first step, we measured chloride concentrations in artificially-maintained brain slices using our 'classic' approaches. We rapidly discovered that neurons effectively had high concentrations of chloride and that applying bumetanide on the brain slices *in vitro* reduced the concentrations efficiently, as would oxytocin. However, knowing that autism is 'born' *in utero* and that, as explained above, epidemiological studies suggest that the risk of having an autistic child can be increased by numerous complications during childbirth, we wanted to see whether these high rates of chloride were already evident at childbirth. We floated a risky and possibly far-fetched premise: what if this reaction was eliminated in newborns with autism? In fact, oxytocin, which plays an important role in attachment and communication, is released during childbirth and plays a crucial role between the mother and the child in the first hours of life. In addition, the mutation of signals transmitted by the hormone creates a complex syndrome in the animal, which includes autism. However, this does not provide solid enough data for a researcher to happily use as a basis for the hypotheses. Nevertheless, we decided to try it and it was a real revelation: the type of surprise that justifies an arduous life of research.

Indeed, in our two animal models, chloride concentrations are high from birth. In other words, the dramatic fall in chloride during birth that we observed in age-matched naïve mice does not happen, the brain somehow zaps it; chloride level remains high and the GABA is excitatory before as well as after birth, while networks generate activities that will disrupt these crucial first moments of life (Tyzio et al., 2014). Thus, there is a greater susceptibility to hypoxic accidents and other damages that explain the epidemiological data and a greater sensibility to pain, which we test and demonstrate (Mazzuca et al., 2011). In addition, all of this is reduced by oxytocin, showing how important this reaction is during birth and the crucial decrease in chloride. It is therefore not surprising that 20 to 30% of autistic children are also epileptic and 60% have abnormal EEG tracings. These observations certainly do not prove that human chloride concentrations are high but confirm and consolidate the general hypothesis. They also illustrate well the consubstantial link between fundamental and applied research.

If the chloride concentrations are high during birth and this is later linked with autistic manifestations, can we not reduce them by restoring lower concentrations of chloride during birth? We sought to test this assumption. Mice mothers were subjected to water containing the diuretic for a period of 24 hours from the eve of the presumed birth. Subsequently, the descendants who had only been exposed to bumetanide for a couple of hours during their birth were tested for chloride concentrations as well as cerebral activities and behavioural traits. We noticed that not only did the treatment restore the concentrations of psychological chloride during birth but did so for many weeks after as well (Tyzio et al., 2014). Psychological cerebral activities and social behaviours are restored, and this is the case in the adult animal too. In other words, the concentrations of chloride during birth, and thus the polarity of GABA during labour, exert long-term effects on the pathogenesis of the illness. For the first time, these observations demonstrate that an illness, including when it is triggered by a genetic mutation, can be treated from birth by a substance, leading to long-term effects in descendants once they have reached adulthood. Particularly astonishing, this procedure also improves electrical activities and the behaviour of an X-fragile mouse, in which the syndrome was produced by a genetic mutation. In other words, even when a genetic mutation perturbs the maturation during the embryonic stage, it is still possible to intervene during birth to reduce the consequences, including once they become adults. It is therefore a long-term effect, with birth being the moment that can either mark the development of a genetic mutation or reduce its effects.

It is evident that the relation between birth conditions and harm during labour suggested by the epidemiological data is also confirmed by our observations. It is clearly important that, to develop our understanding and treatment of autism, we must better understand cerebral maturation and the mechanisms of birth. There remains a need to understand the nature of the mechanisms that link these phenomena, and a hypothesis that indicates birth as a stress that can produce a kind of electroshock that is sometimes beneficial to defective cerebral activities during maturation, reducing harmful after-effects. In any case, this convergence that is rarely observed at this data point in mice and humans opens numerous new avenues of study.

These observations stress the importance of child birth in the pathogenesis of autism. In more recent studies, we made yet another major observation that reinforces the importance of intrauterine events and birth in autism. A fundamental question that curiously has not been investigated is the preparation of the embryo's brain to birth. Considering the complex chains of events that must occur within seconds and minutes, somehow the brain must prepare itself and enable certain networks to be able to resume their new functions rapidly. This is readily illustrated by respiratory functions. To shift from an aqueous medium to an aerobic one implies profound alterations. We now know for instance that the amazing high levels of stress molecules released by the newborn at birth are precisely aimed at allowing the classical respiration occurring once out. We decided to compare 3D maps of the brain shortly before and after birth to gain further information on this issue. Indeed, this type of approach can hardly be performed in humans – meaning functional imaging a few minutes before and after birth is of course not feasible. Indirect observations suggest that the volume of the brain increases as expected *in utero* but this increase is slowed down during the third trimester of gestation. This was obtained by comparing the brain volumes in preterm babies all the way from babies born around the 22nd week of gestation to presumed time of birth. This suggests that growth is halted perhaps in order to avoid growth during a complex and vulnerable period. Indeed, in our naïve rats, the 3D brain volumes as that of major structures remained unchanged 24 hours before birth and the day of birth. In contrast, the volume of "autistic" rat brains was increased during birth as that of major brain structures (Cloarec et al., 2019). Furthermore, reconstructing individual neurons confirmed that neurons actually grow during delivery and birth. Interestingly, the brain of children and adolescents are often bigger than age matched naïve ones, this study suggests that the difference stems already *in utero* and at birth. Amazingly, maternal administration of bumetanide during that same period abolished this growth, the brains of autistic rats at birth were not different from one day earlier. Therefore, neurons actually grow during labour and birth in autism but not in age matched naïve animals. This important conclusion implies that somehow the stop order that prepares the brain to birth is not operative in autism.

Other *in utero* conditions are also associated with autism in humans and experimental animals. Indeed, it is well known that a variety of diseases during pregnancy can be deleterious to the fetus including viral and microbial insults such as Maternal Immune Activation (MIA). It is known that this is mediated by an early activation of the immune system leading to an inflammation and the release of all sort of toxins that impact the developmental sequence. Experiments performed initially by a US group (directed by the late P. Patterson (Patterson, 2011)) showed that drugs that mimic this inflammation do impact the brain with a variety of developmental disorders in the offspring. More recently, an elegant study showed that MIA exerts its deleterious effect by a dual action: the release of inflammation molecules associated with the activation of certain types of bacteria in the microbiota. These two actions affect directly the construction of the neocortex, as blocking either of these two phenomena also blocks the cortical malformation. Interestingly, stimulating these malformed regions reproduced the electrical signature of the syndrome, indicating that the aberrant cortex is responsible for these effects, albeit not directly, but via the earlier activation of the microbiota and the immune system. We are dealing here therefore with a vivid illustration of how *in utero* insults impact a variety of biological functions altering brain developmental sequences that are the final common cause of neurological and psychiatric disorders. This complex link is not readily compatible with the simplistic genetic view of these disorders as the intermediary steps abolish the direct link between the triggering cause – a genetic mutation – and the final outcome-a disease.

We repeated these experiments asking if the birth process was immediately and shortly after birth impacted by MIA. We found that the entire process was affected with excitatory actions of GABA at birth following MIA (Chiesa et al., 2018). Other investigations suggest that oxytocin signals are instrumental, as social communication, notably between the mother and the baby, is deficient when oxytocin signals are deficient. In experimental conditions, blocking oxytocin signals at birth aggravates stress and social interactions, suggesting that oxytocin plays an anti-stress role by reducing its effects during a crucial moment. In fact, clinical trials are being conducted to investigate whether intranasal administration of oxytocin attenuates autism, underlining its importance.

To conclude, using the diuretic as a treatment for a restrained but crucial period of time appears to erase some signs of autism for rodents. It is very unusual for clinical and experimental data link together to validate a concept and a treatment. These results validate our hypothesis, confirming the therapeutic possibilities of bumetanide, but also, as is often the case, it introduces major questions regarding treatment, the role of labour, vaginal and C-section delivery being relevant to a whole host of public health issues.

5. On the importance of early diagnosis

Autism can be detected during the first year of life by good clinical observation and people alert to what are often subtle signs. This still remains very difficult and some children who are diagnosed at that age may have no signs of autism when they reach five years of age. However, we know that the first years of life are those when the brain is the most malleable, the most 'plastic', when it can change the most. It is therefore important, if we want to increase the brain's chances of developing in the best possible way with regards to its environment, to determine as fast as possible whether something does not seem to be going right and to attempt to remedy any difficulties by allowing specialised teams who can propose a treatment. A number of strategies are starting to emerge in English-speaking countries as well as in France. One of them is the M-CHAT questionnaire, which uses just twenty-three questions to determine the existence of early signs of autism, usually around the age of two. We need to find a compromise between attempting early diagnoses, which have weak predictive value, and wanting to intervene quickly at the ages when neural networks are building themselves and when we can still rehabilitate certain functions – or at the very least minimise the impact of developmental issues.

Already, in very young children who will later be diagnosed with autism, eye-tracking studies have shown us that we can observe anomalies in their ability to read faces and an intensified interest in geometric shapes compared to social stimuli. The study of visual exploration associated with behavioural questionnaires is a promising road to pursue when attempting to detect early signs and to handle autism at the earliest opportunity.

Among the various care programmes, some have undergone stringent evaluation, which has allowed us to determine their effectiveness. One of these, the 'Early Start' programme from Denver, which is based on emotional sharing and joint attention and imitation, seems one of the most promising. By prompting the children with social motivation, the programme acts on the neurophysiological parts of the brain that are involved in the perception of emotions and in social interactions, which we know to be anomalous is autistic people. Other studies clearly show that the treatment would be even more efficient if it undergone during the early phases of development. This confirms the importance of an early diagnosis in order to start such treatments as soon as possible. These treatments are aimed at preventing the disordered brain activities from cumulating and preventing communication difficulties from consolidating over time.

Experimental data plainly establish that the pathogenesis of autism happens early, which highlights the important role of childbirth and the effectiveness of a quasi-preventative diuretic treatment administered at birth. These observations confirm the importance of high concentrations of chloride in autism and the important interaction between oxytocin and the diuretic. Given that these two molecules have been suggested as effective in their treatment of autism, we now know the importance of chloride concentrations, which are targeted by these two agents. Moreover, the disorder's early onset and its negative cumulative effect, with its exacerbated electrical activity that will make it harder to repair the deficits as time wears on, especially with regards to communication, make early treatment all the more important.

On a more general note, our data suggest that treating autism in the same way that we treat a headache with aspirin is improbable. Given the alteration of brain connections and the way autism affects the construction of the brain *in utero*, it is better to aim for a more modest goal by seeking to prevent the aggravation of symptoms. Actually, a treatment like the one that we are proposing should ultimately make it easier to introduce the child into their school and parental environment, so that they can learn to communicate and integrate in society as early as possible. It is probable that the combination of a treatment like the one that we are proposing and a behavioural therapeutic approach will allow for a better integration and, if this combination is employed early enough, a possible healing of the disorder, again underlining the importance of an early diagnosis and early treatment. It is school, the parental environment and society more generally that will cure or in any case reduce the absence of communication and isolation that characterises autism.

Our publications and the associated press coverage have also led to many requests from parents of autistic children or autistic adults that ask for information on the treatment and often query the slow pace of advances in the field. We easily understand the wish of parents to finally find relief for their suffering and that of their children. It is also important to us to explain that advancements like ours are part of the road leading to the discovery of pharmaceutical medication. This road is long and arduous, involving both important research funds and fights against deep-seated conservative attitudes. It also involves clinical trials, which are crucial to proving and consolidating our data. These have been too scarce to allow us to put forward definitive conclusions as to the effectiveness of bumetanide. Nevertheless, several publications from other groups have both confirmed the elevated intracellular chloride in Fragile-X neurons and a behavioural amelioration produced by the diuretic. One of these studies showed that an adolescent girl with autism exhibited an improvement in EEG activity following bumetanide treatment.

6. What about the girls?

It is generally admitted that boys are two to five times more affected than girls with autism – but is this really the case? One has to bear in mind that most of the screening and diagnostic tests for autism were designed and developed with/for boys, and very few girls are diagnosed at early preschool. However, a lot of them appear later, at adolescence, or even much later when they themselves have a child who happens to have autism. Autism in females is underdiagnosed, and or misdiagnosed. Why is this the case?

One important reason is that girls have a very different way to express autism. They are interested in social situations, and they spend a lot of time trying to understand them, by reading books, playing with dolls and imaginary friends, and trying to imitate others. They are masters in the art of camouflage. They have better language and communication skills than boys, and all this together often lets them go unnoticed until adolescence, where often everything falls apart, because social demands become more complex and they experience more and more difficulties making and maintaining friends. And this is when they start expressing their autism under the form of eating disorders, obsessive compulsive disorders, anxiety, depression, and can even get diagnosed with personality disorders – when the actual underlying cause is in fact autism, and all these manifestations are co-morbidities and or consequences of their condition. Women with autism and a normal IQ become increasingly affected by social difficulties as they become older, a lot of them suffer from abuse that can be emotional, financial and/or sexual, and in consequence an alarming number have suicidal thoughts or attempts suicide (Holliday Willey, 2011, 2014).

There is not enough research done on girls and women with autism, and we need to better understand what the differences are in neuronal and endocrine pathways that make females with autism behave in such a distinct way from males with autism, even though they share the difficulties in communication and social interactions, and the oversensitivity to many physical stimuli including light, sound, touch, etc. Where does their extremely developed capacity for camouflaging come from? Do they have a specific endocrine phenotype? Does oxytocin play a specific role? Do they suffer from more difficulties than males with autism in the perception of threat, that would make them more vulnerable to abuse? We hope that research in the next years will help us answer these crucial questions, and that not only earlier diagnosis will become more common, but also specific strategies will be put in place to specifically support girls and women with autism to navigate through our world without suffering as much as they often do.

V

PROJECT AND PROGRAMME

1. Publishing results

With results like these, which centre on both fundamental science and a suggestion for a new treatment, all that is left for us to do is to publish them and to have them accepted by the community of scientists and clinicians. Particularly important is persuading public authorities of the need to develop this medicine and to grant it market authorisation.

The crucial step in all scientific work is the publication in peer-reviewed journals. In theory, the idea is an excellent one. We submit our article to a journal, which picks two or more experts relevant to the paper's field of study and gives them the paper, on an anonymous basis, for them to evaluate. These experts, usually called referees, will critique (with varying degree of strictness), its methodology, the quality of the results, and the validity of the findings. This system allows in principle for objectivity to be safeguarded and anonymity prevents backlashes against the paper's authors, who will in turn have to critique the criticism they have received. But the system nevertheless suffers from serious contradictions and questionable consequences. The stakes are high. The evaluation and the financing of research are totally dependent on publication and on the journals in which the work is published. We are subject to a real Michelin Guide that holds the power to dispense life or death on laboratories. Journals that are considered prestigious (*Nature* and *Science*, to name the most well-known) receive hundreds of submissions daily. They must keep a few and refuse the rest. Naturally, the pre-selection is ruthless. Editors will have to decide who deserves to pass to the next stage in a few minutes, just on the basis of the title, the summary, and, of course, the laboratory. Consequently, major discoveries go out of the window, to the benefit of mediocre work that is well written and 'sexier'. These journals decide the politics of research in France and elsewhere, because the fashion of evaluating everything in the mode of ratings agencies has taken over the world of research. This in turn creates difficult economic conditions and increased competition, which favours consensus and safe, fashionable topics that are sure to pass this crucial first step. This conformity is probably due to a most regrettable securitisation of research and the pursuit of knowledge. We quickly saw the consequences of this for autism.

A double-blind randomised clinical trial conducted according to the rules that demonstrates a new treatment for autism should, we believe, not cause any problems. It is a common disorder, a sensitive public opinion issue and, in addition, as of now without valid treatment. We were wrong. It must be said that to pretend to treat such a disorder with a diuretic is accepted with difficulty by genetic experts as well as by psychoanalysts and psychiatrists. In their defence, it must be said that, with complex disorders, experts are not always agreed on the best methods with which to measure improvement. This uncertainty, the hesitations of large international journals, which sometimes publish miracle cures before retracting them, the competition between groups and the economic situation, which worsens these challenges, does not do much for risk-taking. The paper is finally accepted for publication and, as predicted, it generates press conferences and significant public interest, through television, radio and newspaper interviews… An exercise to which we graciously submit ourselves. They also quickly generate, as we had expected, a long list of requests from parents who would like to participate in the next clinical trial. Things will now be easier for our future experimental work; it will quickly be accepted by these so-called prestigious publications!

2. Developments in medication: the battle is only just starting

We have often said that developing a drug is a long and costly process, made so by regulators, who want to avoid the flops that often follow new treatments. The road is scattered with make-or-break steps that must be overcome. Investors must also be convinced that the venture will be profitable, even if the molecule we are depending on is already on the market. The marketing of a new treatment can cost up to a few hundred million euros. In the case of bumetanide, a repositioning of an existing molecule, only a few tens of millions are needed. But, because it is a generic drug, securing financing will be much more difficult. Investors like having patents on new molecules because profits from these are colossal, as opposed to a utility patent that protects a new use of a molecule already available on the market. With a diuretic, however, we are dealing with a generic molecule that has been on the market for four decades and without much return on investment. Indeed, with the utility patent, where we are patenting the mechanism and not the molecule, competitors and counterfeit is more likely. The existence of the molecule for one medical condition will prohibit its prescription for another, but this can always be bypassed. Manufacturing and then exploiting such molecules raises risks. This illustrates one of the problems of developing new molecules, it is not enough to have a molecule that has an effect, or even cures, it must also be profitable. Luckily, we were sponsored by the Simons Foundation Autism Research Initiative, which trusted that our observations might pave the way to novel treatments and invested in the company. We were also backed by the French Bettencourt–Schuller Foundation, which deemed it important to help the experimental, non-directly profitable parts of our research on the alteration of neuronal activity in autism and bumetanide treatment.

The complications raised by health authorities involved in such decisions are ludicrous… We quickly realised that Europe does not really exist. Let's start with the French authorities. Warm welcome, long discussions on the steps to follow. Then, concerning Europe, we must fill in a detailed, hundred-page report on everything: the molecule that will be administered, how it will be administered, literature data on its tolerance… We must then send a CD to all forty members of the committee headquartered in London. A preliminary report, put together by three experts chosen by the commission, is positive but asks that the population used in the trial be widened to include children and teens between two and eighteen years of age – we had our work cut out for us! It proved difficult for one because diagnosing a two-year-old is tough and also because, with the breadth of ages covered, heterogeneity might altogether fail the trial. We nevertheless had to attempt it, which required us to carry out a phase IIB trial in which children between two and eighteen years of age would receive different doses in double-blind. It was a 'multicentre trial', which meant that it took place in France and in several other European countries. The trial was completed in spring 2015, before a final phase III on more patients and more participating centres was to be undertaken.

The trials were carried out by a private organisation, Neurochlore, a small company that acquired the utility patent of the molecule for treating autism. It raised many millions of euros and was therefore the clinical trial sponsor. It was predicted that we would finish in mid-2015. We were of course faced with huge demand from parents who wanted to take part in the clinical trials. It is sadly not possible to include all of them as the criteria used to decide who takes part are strict, otherwise the trial can fail. We could not accept children that did not match the rigid criteria imposed by the authorities to ensure a serious and indisputable testing of the treatment's effects. For example, we could not accept autistic children who suffer from epileptic fits, as it could lead to false conclusions (the agent would reduce the number of fits but not autism itself). We could not accept children who were taking other treatments, as stopping these might have dangerous repercussions. Essentially, we were tirelessly repeating that this stage could not be poorly carried out, as then delay would be inevitable, and could lead to the treatment being abandonment.

The convergence between our clinical observations, brain imaging, and our experimental work tended to validate our hypothesis and confirm the usefulness and therapeutic promise of bumetanide. This important point reassured us in our belief that we were on the right route. We will now have to understand how the chloride concentrations were reached (which biochemical pathway?), and in what similar circumstances did such disorders occur, potentially allowing us to widen our approach to include other disorders. It is also necessary to undertake experimental studies on the role of caesarean birth and the role of oxytocin. On the clinical front, and in parallel with the clinical trials, we must determine whether sensory responses, which we know are heightened in autistic children, are sensitive to bumetanide. We also need to address the kinds of syndrome that are best improved and best corrected by the drug, by using a larger number of patients. Finally, with regards to imagery, we will have to explore the effects of bumetanide on different areas of the brain also using a wider population sample. The good news is that our phase IIB trial also showed a significant attenuation in autism's major symptoms following bumetanide treatment. We are therefore in a better position and have the necessary funds to proceed to the last phase, III.

3. Phase III has started

After many discussions with European health authorities, a final phase III protocol was approved. It consists in 1 year inclusions – a 6-month double-blind and 6 months' open treatment for all, the argument being that the authorities wanted to have children treated 1 year total to determine the efficacy and the side effects after 1 year of treatment. The success or failure is determined after 6 months of treatment (or placebo). 400 children 2 to 18 years old thus covering the entire paediatric population have to be recruited in over 40 centres in 7 EU countries (in fact, there were 2 independent trials, one on 2-7 years old and another one on 7-18 years old) . This is a complex trial as such long periods can be associated with more drop outs and as these are counted as having the initial CARS values, they necessarily reduce the change of statistically significant differences between treated and placebo. A complex long negotiation with a French pharma enabled the trial to be financed and results were expected by the end of 2021 and a drug in the market at best by the end of 2023. If successful, this will be an illustration of the importance of combining basic and clinical observations and perhaps most importantly following our own intuition in spite of the limited initial evidence to substantiate it.

Addendum

In the period separating the writing and publication of this book and 2023, we have advanced in oru efforts with positive and negative outcomes that are summarized below.

i) A failure

The final phase 3 trial was performed (2019-2022) with negative results. There was no significant difference between children treated with Bumetanide and placebo. This situation is not unprecedented, all large phase 3 performed to treat Neurodevelopmental disorders failed. This is in part due to the heterogeneity of Autism and other developmental disorders. Nevertheless, this failure – contrasting with many posiyive phase 2 trials performed during this period – does not imply necessarily the end of the story and the abandon of bumetanide. Indeed, two dutch and Chinese studies showed that EEG and immunological measures can identify children who will respond positively to Bumetanide. This is important considering the fact that if bumetanide is efficient to attenuate autism in say 25-30% of children, it remains a significant tool to attenuate the burden to many children and their parents considering the lack of alternative. We have recently used Machine Learning to re-examine the data collected in the phase 3 and are identifying subpopulations of responders. This does not imply that Bumetanide will be present in pharmacies to treat autism as European and USA agencies will demand a new phase 3 trial and we will not succeed to raise the funds required after the failure of phase 3. Nevertheless, the information available will be unable to use the generic drug under tha control of treating doctors.

ii) A success

If Autism is born in utero, we should be able to identify at birth babies who will be autistic later. This has major implications not only to enable early use of psycho-educative tools-shown to be more efficient when initiated early- but also to complement psychiatric diagnosis with solid biological features. We have tested this hypothesis by collecting a posteriori all maternity data of children who were diagnosed with autism a few years later. These parameters were compared to those of Neurotypic children born in the same maternity and conditions. With machine Learning program, we can identify at birth almost half the autistic children and all the neurotypic children. Impacting parameters are for some expected – bacterial or viral infections during maternity – but for many unexpected- length of the femur bone 2nd trimester or head now position earlier than in Neurotypic foetuses. Interestingly, the Cephalic Perimeter is bigger shortly before birth in future children with Autism than future neurotypic ones (Caly et al, 2021). We are now proceeding with larger a posteriori et a priori data in order to validate these observations.

VI

Conceptual Questions and Criticisms of the Genocentric Approach

Our work raises general conceptual issues regarding autism and other brain disorders. We will address these by way of a conclusion to this essay. We will start our journey with a discussion on brain developmental disorder and the concepts that emerge from our work on autism and on other disorders caused by a faulty construction of the brain. We will then end on what we deem to be the excessive hopes placed in genetics and gene therapy.

1. The construction programme does not always go as planned

What is happening when, for one reason or another, the programme is poorly executed? It must be remembered that more than 80% of genes are in operation as the brain is being built and that, therefore, a mutation in any of these genes can cause damage long before birth. A good number of the genetic mutations involved in brain malformations influence proliferation, migration, and differentiation, essentially affecting most of the crucial phases of brain creation. Classifying these mutations and the clinical and morphological damage they cause improves our diagnostic abilities.

When a mutation is causally linked to the expression of a disorder, identifying the mutation enables a reliable diagnosis to be made even before it is possible to do so clinically. The presence of certain mutations can therefore be translated into the absence of certain brain structures and even into gigantic cortical neurons and epileptic fits, mental retardation and other grave consequences. Often, but not always, these mutations can manifest themselves in modifications of the brain's architectural makeup.

Brain imaging can therefore allow us to identify malformations and therefore better diagnose illnesses. The development of imagery techniques has indeed meant that we have a better understanding of the frequency of these malformations and their role in a number of disorders. Today, we deem that 30% of severe precocious epilepsy is due to brain malformations, whilst this number was just anecdotal a few years ago. This is a direct consequence of the improvement of these techniques, which allow us to see and therefore understand these disorders in greater detail. It is likely that this number will increase and that brain malformations will be discovered in relation to very many disorders in the future.

Imagery's role in diagnosis and treatment is well illustrated by the mutation that causes the formation of a double cortex. This mutation involves a protein appropriately named 'doublecortin'. It is a gene that, when it mutates, causes the ossification of neurons. These neurons then migrate with difficulty, ending up stuck in the bottom layers of the cortex. By accumulation, they end up forming of a 'double cortex', a cortex that is not positioned correctly depth-wise. This will prevent the healthy cortex from functioning properly, causing drug-resistant epileptic fits, mental retardation and an array of debilitating repercussions. Imagery allows us to identify and locate the double cortex, ultimately making it accessible for removal. Curative surgical resection of the diseased tissue prevents epileptic fits and their after-effects. If carried out early, and by a nimble-fingered surgeon, this surgery can be a real miracle as it will enable future development that is as harmonious as possible for the child. Sadly, the results are much poorer, and often null, if the procedure is undertaken later when the circuits have already matured.

To conclude, a great number of disorders are 'born' early. They can alter one or many of the steps involved in the construction of the brain: an excessive proliferation or indeed a limited one, the formation of clumps of displaced cells or anomalous connections between neurons, or the creation of flawed cerebral sulci. Recent studies performed both post mortem and with live imaging indeed showed important alterations in cortical construction in children and adults with autism. These alterations point to an intrauterine origin when these cortices are formed. All these defects in the construction of the brain are persistent signatures alerting us to deficiencies. These malformations will be translated into clinical syndromes, the acuteness of which is dependent on the malformation's own severity. The malformations and their repercussions are pathologies because of the way the programme has been badly executed, leading to the creation of displaced neurons and faulty connections, which will generate activity that disturbs the brain's functioning. There can be a very long delay between the initial cause (the genetic mutation *in utero*) and its clinical manifestation. The correct explanation is sometimes given by clinical observations. For example, when there have been periods of hypoxia-ischemia during a difficult birth, the effects are not immediate on the baby. Epileptic fits may manifest themselves only decades later. Brain imaging will show that that there has been a degeneration of the hippocampus caused by the initial hypoxic-ischaemic episode. The immature brain can therefore work normally after that initial episode but encounter difficulties later on. Indeed, experimental data show that, paradoxically, young neurons are infinitely more resistant to an absence of oxygen than adult neurons, especially during birth. Lucky that it is so as, if not, we would certainly not be here to tell this story given the huge stress we undergo at birth. When the lack of oxygen is over a long period of time, however, consequences are inevitable. In the most severe cases, they immediately lead to cerebral palsy or, if less severe, to epileptic fits later on. All complications in the construction of the brain are here, present at once in a great resistance and a great fragility with regards to what can upend the programme. These observations allow us to better understand why dating the start of a disorder at its first clinical symptoms is not correct. Of course, symptoms can manifest themselves immediately with certain mutations or with severe injury. But the faults in the programming are often translated into preclinical signs, with few or no actual clinical signs being manifested. They will set a scene favourable for repercussions and greater vulnerability to events that would usually be insignificant. The disorder will then evolve progressively, expressing itself only once these malformations become problematic and preventing other circuits from working properly. These preliminary effects will ultimately multiply during the crucial steps in childhood and sometimes adolescence, preventing proper development. There are therefore both direct and collateral effects. The better the importance, and the difficulty, of early detection of these precursory signs of the future disorder becomes clearer.

This distinction between initial causes of a disorder and its expression does not only apply to early-onset disorders. Data suggest that premonitory symptoms precede clinical ones for late-onset disorders, such as Parkinson's and Alzheimer's. An American team used brain imagery to study patients suffering from Huntington's chorea, a monogenic disorder where the mutation is causally linked to the disorder. The researchers showed that brain malformations are present in the brain years before the first signs of the disorder are expressed. Early diagnosis can also raise ethical problems when there are no therapeutic treatments, as is the case for Huntington's chorea. We do not have the expertise to take part this debate but optimism, rigour, and understanding the evolution of a disorder will allow us one day to treat it early. In any case, burying our heads in the sand will not allow us to progress.

2. "Neuroarcheology", or the search for presymptomatic signs of neurological disorders

If mutations or environmental issues can cause malformations whilst often expressing themselves later on, it becomes urgent for us to better understand how these malformations act early and modify the programme. We have proposed a concept, 'neuroarcheology', to refer to the presence of pre-symptomatic signs resulting from these early malformations that flag up disorders to come (Ben-Ari, 2008). These signs can be architectural (such as the presence of a double cortex detected using an MRI scan) or electric (such as specific electric discharge patterns generated by displaced neurons) and prevent the brain's construction and harmonious functioning. A bit like an archaeologist, we search within malformations for the events that they have caused. In analogy, we can now readily determine why and how a given building collapsed. A key question is then posed: if the electrical activity of a neuron is modified by the programme's realisation, could it be that electric activity also holds a sign of this delay?

To test this hypothesis, we used rodents with mutations that cause malformations in humans and are expressed *in utero*. We can then record the electrical activity of the displaced neurons at different stages of the maturation process and determine their properties. The transfection of the doublecortin, which causes the formation of a double cortex in humans, does so as well in the animal: a cluster of cells appears at the depth of the cortex, where there should not usually be one. Recording the neurons that remain there shows us that they keep their immature properties even when the adult stage is reached. Everything happens as if the neurons that do not connect or migrate properly stay stuck in an immature state, emitting electrical signals that correspond to that phase. There is therefore an electrical signature on top of the architectural one of the displaced neurons. Similar observations were made with other mutations involved in different disorders. Actually, a large collection of genetic mutations was expressed *in utero* in the rodent, leading to malformations. Displaced or badly connected neurons were then seen to exhibit particular properties. These observations opened up an important therapeutic perspective. If a displaced neuron generates an immature current at a later stage that it is not meant to generate, we can imagine selectively blocking harmful currents using selective antagonists, which act against these currents. This is not a far-fetched or illusory idea; there are already many molecules with such properties that are commonly used by scientists to study brain maturation. Trials are also underway to develop such a strategy, notably with regards to epilepsy. Our approach for autism illustrates this well. Chloride concentrations are high *in utero* and remain so in the autistic brain, as opposed to the neurotypical brain. Bumetanide indeed has no effect on healthy adult neurons, which have low chloride concentrations, but it reduces the high concentrations present in the autistic brain.

In sum, a good number of disorders are born early but are expressed much later on. The causes of these disorders will alter the proper development of the genetic programme, sometimes causing clinical signs much later on. The neurons that suffered during this event remain stuck at an immature stage, leaving a signature from the maturation phase of when the cessation happened. Therapeutic treatments are possible, which are based on the selective blocking of the activities generated by these immature neurons in the adult brain. The concept of neuroarcheology proposes that there are architectural and/or electrical traces, the relics of a programme that was not executed correctly. This is illustrated by our work on autism and our proposal of treating it with a diuretic that acts on the high chloride concentrations observed in immature neurons and in pathological conditions. If confirmed, this will heavily impact our understanding of the links between the clinical manifestation of cerebral disorders and their origin stressing the importance of studying brain development in order to treat them.

3. Genetic reductionism's takeover bid for autism

It cannot be contested that the genetic revolution allowed for considerable advances in many fields, from population genetics and evolution to biology in general and neurobiology in particular. We can get sure-fire diagnoses when we identify monogenic mutations (mutations where a single gene is necessary and sufficient for causing the disorder). In some cases, it can give hope for an effective therapy, as with some cancers or leukaemia. Diagnosis is a huge relief for patients and their families: the pain is given a name, and they can inform themselves, come together with other families, and create associations. In short, they are not isolated, not alone in the face of adversity. Knowing what protein or biological pathway causes the disorder often opens up important opportunities for intervening at one of the points in the chain that caused the deficiency.

Yet this correction is rarely translated by a direct correction of the defective gene, by gene therapy, that is. This approach remains wishful thinking for the time being and has only been tested successfully in only two disorders. In other words, identifying a mutation, including for monogenic disorders, does not guarantee the existence of a therapy. Many decades after having identified the mutations responsible for cystic fibrosis or Duchenne muscular dystrophy, we are still unarmed against them. There are many obstacles that must be overcome to understand the biological reaction pathways caused by a mutation, from the heterogeneity of cell components to the difficulty of introducing in a targeted manner the 'right' gene where it is required, to the need to avoid dangerous consequences of genetic manipulation.

The situation is much more complicated and can become almost impossible when we are faced with complex disorders, where tens if not hundreds of mutations are responsible for the disorder and in particular with complex psychiatric symptoms. Unfortunately, most neurological and psychiatric disorders have a polygenic cause. A mutation can be at the root of many disorders and many mutations can cause the same disorder, preventing an easy diagnosis based on the identification of one mutation. It is as if we have too many mutations for one disorder and too many disorders for the same mutation. The early-onset of a disorder and its impact on mutations will also cause a chain of events that complicates matters further as correcting the situation *in utero* (which is the only option to prevent the event) is nigh impossible. Moreover, the heterogeneity of nerve cells, the extraordinary ability to re-adapt and modify neural networks, and the bearing electrical activity has on the functioning of these groups on in addition to their inaccessibility, highlights the difficulty of reasoning in causal terms. However, in spite of these limitations, we can promise miracles daily thanks to the genetic revolution. Along the way, a generation of young researchers has been sacrificed on the altar of the 'all-genetics'. The youth will be trained wherever there is a future, where they can be published in prestigious journals, where they can be recruited and then build a promising career. The establishment has clearly chosen its camp: prestigious journals, popular newspapers… All sing praises to this revolution. Telethon-style fundraisers exemplify this infatuation. However, three to four decades after disorder-causing mutations were identified, like that of Huntington's chorea, we are far from having even the slightest idea as to a possible treatment. This shows us the kind of cul-de-sac we find ourselves in after dedicating ourselves to an approach that exclusively focuses on and privileges genetics.

The decisive next step is 'post-genetics', which starts with the gene and tries to understand the chain of events that follows it. To better understand and treat these disorders, it is paramount that we understand why and in particular how these mutations have caused the formation of atypical neural networks. It is a long-winded approach that requires the coordinated efforts of physiologists, pharmacologists, anatomists, anatomo-pathologists, and biochemists to dissect the effects of these initial mutations. The problem is that fashion has moved on from there and these fields are now considered dated. We are finally starting to understand these difficulties and promises are few and far between, generally uttered by certain witch doctors or perhaps in Lourdes for those who believe in miracles…

We clearly cannot dissociate environmental genes/brain activity during brain development, as they work together in series and not in parallel. One impacts and the other corrects, and this happens from the earliest stages. Nothing is set in stone, no biological reaction operates without a retroactive control, and this is precisely what electrical activity does by checking at each moment that everything is going according to plan. English researchers recently published a study that looked at the probability of the autism phenotype being expressed in homozygous twins as a function of the geographic location of where they lived in the UK. In theory, the expression of the phenotype should be independent from the environment. However, the probability of the expression of the disorder differed whether the twins lived in London, Birmingham or Glasgow. In addition, the socio-economic background had an effect, where there was a difference between underprivileged areas and ones that were more privileged. This issue hints at the role fashions play in science. Fashions have existed throughout science's history: electrophysiology had its moment, as did anatomy or behavioural sciences. These lasted a certain amount of time before being replaced by others, which were deemed to better answer the questions of their times. Technology is indeed never far away, given that the tools it provides are the basis of significant advances. It allows researchers to shake up contemporary conceptual frameworks. We are left with the fact that the genetic revolution has firmly established itself in the scientific landscape for a while to come. The main reason is that the genetic language encompasses our times perfectly. The modern world is a hurried one. Complex issues need to be summed up in a formula, preferably as a number – a bit like what we see with ratings agencies. Genetics plays the game well: it is easier to say that such-and-such disorder is caused by the replacement of a letter by another than to enter into complex discussions of pH, acidity or ionic equilibria. We would be painting an incomplete picture if we did not say that identifying mutations has allowed us to generate GMOs, mice in which these genes are mutated so we can study the consequences. These tools are very useful, providing a means that is of course complex and that must be handled with care, but that allows us to study the role a given protein has on the brain's functioning. These studies have provided a fount of data that ultimately allow us to explore the mechanisms that are actually known to exist in a good number of pathologies, such as brain inhibition, synaptic plasticity, or the functioning of certain neural networks. By using these GMOs, we have been able to further the study of brain malfunctions and to show that brain inhibition is affected, in particular with regards to the equilibrium between excitation and inhibition. This has also provided an explanation for why up to a quarter of autistic people suffer from epileptic fits. These studies have allowed us to show that particular GABAergic neurons are perhaps involved. However, these neurons are associated with the genesis of specific brain rhythms, gamma rhythms, of forty to eighty cycles per second, which are known for their particular function in the establishment of integrative functions, such as the synchronisation of activities between the two brain hemispheres. These studies have thus opened up interesting new avenues for further work.

4. A critique of gene therapy for treating developmental disorders

Let us imagine a mutation that is involved in psychiatric illnesses. To simplify, let us take the rare case of a disorder caused by a monogenic mutation. The expression of this mutation and the resulting invalidation of the protein that results from it are conditions necessary and sufficient for the expression of the disorder. If this mutation is expressed early, as is often the case, it will affect the construction of the brain to various degrees, culminating in the formation of clusters of displaced and poorly-connected cells, as we have seen. In turn, this will be translated into exacerbated activity that modifies the functioning of the neural networks, creating a chain of events and, later on, a clinical syndrome. Treating this disorder at a late stage by correcting the mutated gene, such as by reintroducing it, has the risk of being ineffective because the disorder is not the same thing as the invalidation of the gene that started off the chain of events but instead is the anomalous activities that were produced by the mutation. Thus, even if we would try to introduce a 'good' gene, which is far from technically possible nowadays, we would prevent the direct causes of the disorder. It is a bit like judging that the crucial phenomenon after a car crash caused by a ruptured tyre is the tyre itself and not the engine that was destroyed by the accident and want to repair the tyre not the motor. Admittedly, immature neurons have a large degree of 'plasticity' (a term that has been at times distorted), but badly connected neurons are not corrected by a magic plasticity mechanism. We indeed know that with the epileptic fits that follow accidents or diverse injuries, neurons can reconnect. However, this so-called 'reactive' plasticity worsens symptoms, they do not improve them. Of course, this is all the more so when it comes to disorders caused by a number of mutations, where their combined actions will be multiplied by many chains of modifications that alter brain development.

Recent experiments indeed reintroduced a correct double-cortin gene *in utero* in an animal using a conditional technique once the neurons have migrated badly and the animals are epileptic. The introduction of the good gene did correct the migration and reduced the epilepsy but only for a handful of days after birth. Such an operation produced no results when conducted several days later. In other words, genetic correction (gene therapy) is possible only during a short early phase that corresponds with the mother's pregnancy, making it impossible to carry out. As the diagnosis is not always certain, we can have the mutation and no symptoms. Introducing the gene *in utero* by targeting certain neurons without triggering the chain of harmful consequences then seems like mission impossible. All things considered, there are strong chances that gene therapy will long remain a false idea, at least for the brain disorders we are addressing here. Genetics nevertheless allows us in rare cases to establish a diagnostic, even if a cure is not possible. This is not without worth as parents are often relieved to know that their child's disorder has been identified and has a name.

Still, in some slow-progressing disorders, experimental data suggest that a part of the deficiency can be corrected by introducing a 'good' gene. For example, with Rett syndrome, which has autistic characteristics, encouraging results from experiments where a mouse is endowed with a conditional mutation in the MecP2 gene, the regulatory gene that is mutated in this disorder. In a way, this technique allows us to switch the mutation on or off at the chosen age and therefore avoid the maturation step and its effect on the disorder's expression. Consequently, we may express the mutation later on or correct it by either expressing or switching the symptoms on/off. A Scottish team has shown that it is possible to produce part of the symptoms by expressing the mutation in the adult stage. In other words, some symptoms of the disorder are not due to a chain of maturation steps but directly due to the mutation, as we can observe them as soon as the mutation is expressed. So gene therapy could be possible but the obstacles outlined above would still have to be cleared – which is far from being the case. The MecP2 protein activates the hundreds of molecules and processes, making it difficult to predict which will be correctable in the future. This disorder is deemed particularly interesting by some experts because early signs actually do exist but they are hard to see. If the symptoms are progressively expressed along a scale of increasing severity, it then stops being a developmental disorder in the proper sense of the term. We need to await more complete work on the MecP2 protein, its role, its actions, and its development before we are truly able to understand the particularities of Rett syndrome. It seems unlikely that the brain is unaffected already at birth in this syndrome and until this has been shown not to be the case, care must be exerted before concluding the developmental factors do not contribute to Rett syndrome.

In conclusion, correcting by introducing a 'good' gene is a rather unlikely option for the majority of brain disorders because the mutation is expressed early and creates a chain of events. Gene therapy is promising for peripheral disorders and cancers but not for an organ as plastic as the brain.

5. The early onset of many disorders causes difficult problems but also has some promise

Dating the start of a disorder does not depend on when the first signs appear. We saw this in the context of the improvement of imagery techniques and determining the onset of epilepsy caused by brain malformations. This dating cannot depend on detection methods as this would make our diagnostic capabilities dependent on technological evolution. It is essential to develop early detection methods for disorders so that we stop depending on the quality of the doctor treating us. Recently, developments in memory testing techniques have brought the dating of Alzheimer's forward by ten years. It is likely that we will see further advances in this direction. Effectively, the dating of disorders cannot depend on technical advances, nor on the quality of the tests, nor on the doctors that use them. Dating must depend on a better understanding of the events that culminate in the expression of a disorder's symptoms, so as to detect precursor signs early on. We call these 'biomarkers'.

It therefore becomes key for us to better understand how the brain mechanisms are led astray by genetic mutations and/or environmental factors. The problem is particularly poignant when it comes to disorders that have an *in utero* cause, as it is especially difficult to develop medicines that both respect the mother's needs and those of the embryo. It is a Catch-22.

Moreover, politics balk at financing research in the environmental effect on pregnancy because of the financial and employment issues it generates. This is a major public interest issue considering the increasingly popular reliance on programmed C-sections, the increase in preterm delivery and inflammation *in utero*, which are to various degrees associated with the increased incidence of autism and other developmental brain disorders. The impact of modern life, stress, and pesticides can readily be added to this gloomy picture. And, of course, the pharmaceutical industry will also not be interested in such work. All this means that sources of funding prefer sensible genetic explanations that, wrongly so, seek not to question environmental factors and seek to relieve politics of any responsibility. Finally, and as an added complication, an early diagnosis does not necessarily indicate the existence of an adequate treatment, which raises ethical questions. Research has nevertheless opened up advances that will usher in new treatment options, of which autism is a striking example. There is little doubt that the impact of modern life with its stress, pollution and tough conditions in many during child bearing and birth stands at the core of the alterations and increase incidence of various disorders including autism. We will have to adapt our research to take into account these factors in spite of the ever- growing trend of dominating modes notably technical innovations.

VII

GENERAL CONCLUSIONS

This book followed the path from the initial concept to the medication, insisting on the process' complexity. We have few theories and constraining data on the mechanisms involved, and evaluating the effectiveness of medical treatment is further complicated by the fact that we are dealing with psychiatric illnesses. Each expert has their own technique that they consider the most trustworthy. In their defence, it must be said that placebo effects play a large role, crippling our ability to determine whether a treatment has a positive effect or not. Administrative and financial difficulties inherent to any enterprise add themselves to the mix, with problems arising when applying for international patents or undertaking clinical trials. Along the way, we have acquired a new profession and have learned to manage areas that have till now been unknown. We are nevertheless left with much: the feedback from the patients and the satisfaction of discovering new scientific concepts, which represent progress in knowledge. Our trio's adventure exemplifies the importance of multidisciplinary work. Meetings of minds not only enrich work and foster success but also strengthen our belief that we are on the right path. We can only regret the conceptual weakness of modern scientific research which, with its methods and financing, pens in research, favouring short-termism and extreme specialisation to the detriment of the all-important need of taking a step back and thinking big.

Marcel Proust: 'The real act of discovery consists not in finding new lands, but in seeing with new eyes'. *Victor Hugo* (when commenting on a man sentenced to death): 'Nature sketched him badly and education did not improve the draft.' Nature (the genetic programme) provides the draft, but education (the environment) transforms it into a complete work – which was not the case for that sentenced man. And as Yehezkel Ben-Ari is fond of saying, 'Discoveries are always made on side roads, not on highways.'

VIII

APPENDICES

1. The neither-nor, or a third way: an article summarising our stance

In an article published in *Le Monde*, 22 February 2012, we summed up the debate as such: 'Treating autism: neither reductionism nor a psychoanalytic ritual!' ('Le traitement de l'autisme: ni réductionnisme ni rituel psychanalytique!')

The epic debates that currently concern the causes of autism will leave anyone unfamiliar with the topic rather perplexed. Ideological conflicts far removed from the medical and biological reality seem to flourish particularly well in autism. Here are a few undeniable facts to clear things up a bit:

Autism is an early-onset disorder, often born during pregnancy

We find more neurons in certain brain regions of autistic children. This cellular proliferation happens exclusively *in utero* in humans. That is irrefutable proof. Autism is a disorder arising from brain development, with anomalous neural networks forming very early on, which make communication in autistic children difficult from their youngest age.

Autism sometimes has a genetic origin but the environment plays a crucial role

We have identified genetic mutations in animals that cause malformations and 'autistic behavioural traits'. These mutations influence the creation of connections between nerve cells and pitch the embryo's brain into a vicious cycle, having deleterious effects on the affected areas.

Epidemiological studies show that there are numerous environmental factors that have a bearing on autism

A Danish study on the correlation between autism and birth complications show that there are more than sixty perinatal factors that are linked to autism: abnormal position of the baby during birth, umbilical/placental complications, foetal distress, injuries or neonatal traumas, multiple births, maternal haemorrhage, summer birth, low birth weight, an embryo small for its gestational age, congenital malformation, nutritional difficulties, neonatal anaemia, ABO incompatibility, or Rhesus disease. The probability of having an autistic child increases when at least two of the factors are combined. Toxins, such as heavy metals and pesticides, also have a bearing on the disorder being expressed. In all, autism is a multifactorial developmental disorder.

Brain malformation is a 'biological' phenomenon – it is not floating in ether and will not be cured by words

To speak of the mother's responsibility and of the wish to solve her relationship with her child goes against what is ultimately a biological situation. Oxytocin, for example, the hormone released during birth and breastfeeding, plays a definite role in the attachment between mother and child. Imagine that this hormone works less well for a particular mother and her child; would we accuse the mother of being responsible for this and attempt to cure a difficult relationship with words rather than with the deficient hormone? We must remember that even the affective aspects that psychoanalysts are so affectionate about essentially have a biological substratum.

Psychoanalysts' pretence that they can cure this disorder with sessions of psychoanalysis does not hold as biology cannot be ignored. The lack of scientific basis in the field and the fact that it relies on the bare minimum of statistical proofs that others are normally compelled to show if they want to develop treatments is simply unacceptable. Moreover, not only is proof of improvement still awaited, the method itself has devastating effects by blaming mothers and by making the child lose time as they are prevented from an education that could allow them to develop and integrate. At the other extreme, genetic reductionism starts with an abusive simplification that, whilst clearing mothers of their responsibilities, does not take sufficient stock of environmental factors. We have identified hundreds of mutations associated with autism, many of which are also at the origin of other neurological disorders. There are therefore many genes for the same disorder and many disorders for the same gene, illustrating the difficulty of diagnosis and gene therapy's illusory quality. We should not be in a situation where a double takeover bid, for the disorder and for parents whose courage deserves huge respect and admiration, is being proposed. The disorder and its treatment pose a serious problem for researchers. It must be addressed pragmatically and seriously, free from *a priori*. Parents often say that the medical takeover of their child's care is difficult for them. This is due on the one hand to the mothers' sense of guilt, which it often fosters, but mainly because it creates a hierarchy of priorities that does not usually take into account the key objectives of autonomy and integration. Parents have often rightly expressed a feeling of having their parental roles taken away from them, of being rendered incapable of making choices for their child.

Courage is required to say that the disorder will not be cured in the way that we are used to, as with an aspirin treating a headache. Different methods already help us improve parents' daily life – that is already a step in the right direction. The squabbling between left and right has no place here, marrying the left with psychoanalysis is as simplistic as pretending that behavioural approaches are necessarily right-wing. Let us start by understanding better how disordered networks are built, how to eventually reduce their dangerous effect on neighbouring networks and especially how to alleviate all this. Only then will we be moving forward. Let us stop promising miracle cures, whether with a gene or a molecule that will erase the after-effects of developmental malformations. It is by blocking anomalous activity using pharmacological tools that the most serious promises are being developed.

We clearly believe that the binary framework for autism needs to be revisited. As with other disorders that are born during the embryonic stage, analysis and potential therapy of these disorders must take into account the initial cause of the neural malformation. This malformation creates a vicious cycle that worsens the consequences and, importantly, often renders this initial cause secondary. Treatment must therefore centre around the functioning of these disordered networks in order to block them. Identifying the earliest phases of the disorder becomes of great importance given our wish to prevent this vicious cycle.

2. Provisional conclusion: we must take into account the crucial role played by the environment in which the brain is formed

Things again get a bit complicated when we study the general factors that can increase the chances of having an autistic child. As we have seen, the Danish meta-analysis showed that a large number of perinatal factors can be linked to autism. None of these factors are sufficient by themselves, but the convergence of two or more of them is causally linked to autism. A double sentence if you will, as the factors' consequences cumulate. The authors of this systematic study do relieve assisted vaginal delivery of responsibility, as well as post-term birth, a high birth weight or a large head circumference.

Other elements that are correlated with the probability of having an autistic child are added to this list of factors, such as toxins, pesticides, or even other factors related to pregnancy that can have adverse effects on brain maturation such as taking some medication like serotonin reuptake inhibitors – the most famous of which is Prozac®. Pregnancy, a dangerous time! A very recent study showed that obesity of the mother during pregnancy is also a risk factor. A plethora of incidents that can intervene during the first phases of life are thus added to the many mutations involved in autism. This convergence of multiform factors and mechanisms that can play a role explains the difficulty that researchers face when studying the causes and therapeutic approaches likely to reduce the consequences. If we add to these the fact that the disorder concerns communication with others and empathy, it becomes clear why autism is at the heart of important societal debates.

IX

REFERENCES

Attwood, T. (2007). *The complete guide to Asperger's syndrome*. Philadelphia, PA: Jessica Kingley Publishers.

Baio, J., Wiggins, L., Christensen, D. L., Maenner, M. J., Daniels, J., Warren, Z., . . . Dowling, N. F. (2018). Prevalence of Autism Spectrum Disorder Among Children Aged 8 Years — Autism and Developmental Disabilities Monitoring Network, 11 Sites, United States, 2014. *CDC MMWR Surveill Summ 2018, 67*, 1-23. doi: http://dx.doi.org/10.15585/mmwr.ss6706a1

Ben-Ari, Y. (2008). Neuro-archaeology: pre-symptomatic architecture and signature of neurological disorders. *Trends Neurosci, 31*(12), 626-636. doi:10.1016/j.tins.2008.09.002

Ben-Ari, Y. (2014). The GABA excitatory/inhibitory developmental sequence: a personal journey. *Neuroscience, 279*, 187-219. doi:10.1016/j.neuroscience.2014.08.001

Ben-Ari, Y. (2015). Is birth a critical period in the pathogenesis of autism spectrum disorders? *Nat Rev Neurosci, 16*(8), 498-505. doi:10.1038/nrn3956

Ben-Ari, Y. (2017). NKCC1 Chloride Importer Antagonists Attenuate Many Neurological and Psychiatric Disorders. *Trends Neurosci*. doi:10.1016/j.tins.2017.07.001

Ben-Ari, Y., Cherubini, E., Corradetti, R., & Gaiarsa, J. L. (1989). Giant synaptic potentials in immature rat CA3 hippocampal neurones. *The Journal of physiology, 416*, 303-325.

Ben-Ari, Y., Gaiarsa, J. L., Tyzio, R., & Khazipov, R. (2007). GABA: a pioneer transmitter that excites immature neurons and generates primitive oscillations. *Physiological reviews, 87*(4), 1215-1284. doi:10.1152/physrev.00017.2006

Ben-Ari, Y., & Spitzer, N. C. (2010). Phenotypic checkpoints regulate neuronal development. *Trends Neurosci, 33*(11), 485-492. doi:S0166-2236(10)00123-2 [pii] 10.1016/j.tins.2010.08.005

Bergqvist, L. L., Katz-Salamon, M., Hertegard, S., Anand, K. J., & Lagercrantz, H. (2009). Mode of delivery modulates physiological and behavioral responses to neonatal pain. *J Perinatol, 29*(1), 44-50. doi:10.1038/jp.2008.129

Brothers, L. (1990). The social brain: a project for integrating primate behaviour and neurophysiology in a new domain. *Concepts Neurosci, 1*, 27-151.

Chiesa, M., Guimond, D., Tyzio, R., Pons-Bennaceur, A., Lozovaya, N., Burnashev, N., . . . Ben-Ari, Y. (2018). Term or Preterm Cesarean Section Delivery Does Not Lead to Long-term Detrimental Consequences in Mice. *Cereb Cortex*. doi:10.1093/cercor/bhy112

Cloarec, R., Riffault, B., Dufour, A., Rabiei, H., Gouty-Colomer, L.-A., Dumon, C., . . . Ben-Ari, Y. (2019). Pyramidal neuron growth and increased hippocampal volume during labor and birth in autism. *Science Advances, 5*(1), eaav0394. doi:10.1126/sciadv.aav0394

Coleman, M., & Gillberg, C. (2012). *The Autisms*. New York: Oxford University Press.

Czech, H. (2018). Hans Asperger, National Socialism, and "race hygiene" in Nazi-era Vienna. *Mol Autism, 9*, 29. doi:10.1186/s13229-018-0208-6

Dalton, K. M., Nacewicz, B. M., Johnstone, T., Schaefer, H. S., Gernsbacher, M. A., Goldsmith, H. H., . . . Davidson, R. J. (2005). Gaze fixation and the neural circuitry of face processing in autism. *Nature Neuroscience, 8*(4), 519-526.

Dimberg, U. (1982). Facial reactions to facial expressions. *Psychophysiology, 19*(6), 643-647.

Fernandez, A., Dumon, C., Guimond, D., Tyzio, R., Bonifazi, P., Lozovaya, N., . . . Ben-Ari, Y. (2018). The GABA Developmental Shift Is Abolished by Maternal Immune Activation Already at Birth. *Cereb Cortex*. doi:10.1093/cercor/bhy279

Galazka, M. A., Asberg Johnels, J., Zurcher, N. R., Hippolyte, L., Lemonnier, E., Billstedt, E., . . . Hadjikhani, N. (2018). Pupillary Contagion in Autism. *Psychol Sci*, 956797618809382. doi:10.1177/0956797618809382

Guillon, Q., Hadjikhani, N., Baduel, S., & Roge, B. (2014). Visual social attention in autism spectrum disorder: insights from eye tracking studies. *Neurosci Biobehav Rev, 42*, 279-297. doi:10.1016/j.neubiorev.2014.03.013

Hadjikhani, N., Åsberg Johnels, J., Lassalle, A., Zürcher, N. R., Hippolyte, L., Gillberg, C., . . . Ben-Ari, Y. (2018). Bumetanide for autism: more eye contact, less amygdala activation. *Sci Rep, 8*(1), 3602. doi:10.1038/s41598-018-21958-x

Hadjikhani, N., Asberg Johnels, J., Zurcher, N. R., Lassalle, A., Guillon, Q., Hippolyte, L., . . . Gillberg, C. (2017). Look me in the eyes: constraining gaze in the eye-region provokes abnormally high subcortical activation in autism. *Sci Rep, 7*, 3163. doi:10.1038/s41598-017-03378-5

Hadjikhani, N., Joseph, R. M., Manoach, D. S., Naik, P., Snyder, J., Dominick, K., . . . de Gelder, B. (2009). Body expressions of emotion do not trigger fear contagion in autism spectrum disorder. *Soc Cogn Affect Neurosci, 4*(1), 70-78. doi:nsn038 [pii] 10.1093/scan/nsn038

Hadjikhani, N., Joseph, R. M., Snyder, J., Chabris, C. F., Clark, J., Steele, S., . . . Tager-Flusberg, H. (2004). Activation of the fusiform gyrus when individuals with autism spectrum disorder view faces. *Neuroimage, 22*(3), 1141-1150.

Hadjikhani, N., Joseph, R. M., Snyder, J., & Tager-Flusberg, H. (2007). Abnormal activation of the social brain during face perception in autism. *Hum Brain Mapp, 28*(5), 441-449.

Hadjikhani, N., Zurcher, N. R., Rogier, O., Hippolyte, L., Lemonnier, E., Ruest, T., . . . Gillberg, C. (2014). Emotional contagion for pain is intact in autism spectrum disorders. *Transl Psychiatry, 4*, e343. doi:10.1038/tp.2013.113

Hadjikhani, N., Zurcher, N. R., Rogier, O., Ruest, T., Hippolyte, L., Ben-Ari, Y., & Lemonnier, E. (2015). Improving emotional face perception in autism with diuretic bumetanide: a proof-of-concept behavioral and functional brain imaging pilot study. *Autism, 19*(2), 149-157. doi:10.1177/1362361313514141

Helt, M. S., Eigsti, I. M., Snyder, P. J., & Fein, D. A. (2010). Contagious yawning in autistic and typical development. *Child Dev, 81*(5), 1620-1631. doi:10.1111/j.1467-8624.2010.01495.x

Holliday Willey, L. (2011). *Safety Skills for Asperger Women: How to Save a Perfectly Good Female Life* Jessica Kingsley Publishers.

Holliday Willey, L. (2014). *Pretending to be Normal: Living with Asperger's Syndrome (Autism Spectrum Disorder) Expanded Edition* Jessica Kingsley Publishers.

Johnson, M. H., Dziurawiec, S., Ellis, H., & Morton, J. (1991). Newborns' preferential tracking of face-like stimuli and its subsequent decline. *Cognition, 40*(1-2), 1-19.

Lagercrantz, H., & Slotkin, T. A. (1986). The "stress" of being born. *Sci Am, 254*(4), 100-107.

Lassalle, A., Asberg Johnels, J., Zurcher, N. R., Hippolyte, L., Billstedt, E., Ward, N., . . . Hadjikhani, N. (2017). Hypersensitivity to low intensity fearful faces in autism when fixation is constrained to the eyes. *Hum Brain Mapp, 38*(12), 5943-5957. doi:10.1002/hbm.23800

Lassalle, A., Zurcher, N. R., Hippolyte, L., Billstedt, E., Porro, C. A., Benuzzi, F., . . . Hadjikhani, N. (2018). Effect of visual stimuli of pain on empathy brain network in people with and without Autism Spectrum Disorder. *Eur J Neurosci, 48*(6), 2333-2342. doi:10.1111/ejn.14138

Lemonnier, E., & Ben-Ari, Y. (2010). The diuretic bumetanide decreases autistic behaviour in five infants treated during 3 months with no side effects. *Acta Paediatr, 99*(12), 1885-1888. doi:APA1933 [pii] 10.1111/j.1651-2227.2010.01933.x

Lemonnier, E., Degrez, C., Phelep, M., Tyzio, R., Josse, F., Grandgeorge, M., . . . Ben-Ari, Y. (2012). A randomised controlled trial of bumetanide in the treatment of autism in children. *Transl Psychiatry, 2*, e202. doi:10.1038/tp.2012.124

Lemonnier, E., Villeneuve, N., Sonie, S., Serret, S., Rosier, A., Roue, M., . . . Ben-Ari, Y. (2017). Effects of bumetanide on neurobehavioral function in children and adolescents with autism spectrum disorders. *Transl Psychiatry, 7*(3), e1056. doi:10.1038/tp.2017.10

Mazzuca, M., Minlebaev, M., Shakirzyanova, A., Tyzio, R., Taccola, G., Janackova, S., . . . Khazipov, R. (2011). Newborn Analgesia Mediated by Oxytocin during Delivery. *Frontiers in cellular neuroscience, 5*, 3. doi:10.3389/fncel.2011.00003

Morris, J. P., Pelphrey, K. A., & McCarthy, G. (2007). Controlled scanpath variation alters fusiform face activation. *Soc Cogn Affect Neurosci, 2*(1), 31-38.

Patterson, P. H. (2011). Maternal infection and immune involvement in autism. *Trends Mol Med, 17*(7), 389-394. doi:10.1016/j.molmed.2011.03.001

Pichot, P. (1986). [DSM-III: the 3d edition of the Diagnostic and Statistical Manual of Mental Disorders from the American Psychiatric Association]. *Rev Neurol (Paris), 142*(5), 489-499.

Reid, V. M., Dunn, K., Young, R. J., Amu, J., Donovan, T., & Reissland, N. (2017). The Human Fetus Preferentially Engages with Face-like Visual Stimuli. *Curr Biol, 27*(12), 1825-1828 e1823. doi:10.1016/j.cub.2017.05.044

Rivera, C., Voipio, J., Payne, J. A., Ruusuvuori, E., Lahtinen, H., Lamsa, K., . . . Kaila, K. (1999). The K+/Cl- co-transporter KCC2 renders GABA hyperpolarizing during neuronal maturation. *Nature, 397*(6716), 251-255. doi:10.1038/16697

Rizzolatti, G., & Fabbri-Destro, M. (2010). Mirror neurons: from discovery to autism. *Exp Brain Res, 200*(3-4), 223-237. doi:10.1007/s00221-009-2002-3

Robison, J. E. (2008). *Look Me in the Eye: My Life with Asperger's*: Three Rivers Press.

Tyzio, R., Cossart, R., Khalilov, I., Minlebaev, M., Hubner, C. A., Represa, A., . . . Khazipov, R. (2006). Maternal oxytocin triggers a transient inhibitory switch in GABA signaling in the fetal brain during delivery. *Science, 314*(5806), 1788-1792. doi:10.1126/science.1133212

Tyzio, R., Nardou, R., Ferrari, D. C., Tsintsadze, T., Shahrokhi, A., Eftekhari, S., . . . Ben-Ari, Y. (2014). Oxytocin-mediated GABA inhibition during delivery attenuates autism pathogenesis in rodent offspring. *Science, 343*(6171), 675-679. doi:10.1126/science.1247190

Wang, D. D., & Kriegstein, A. R. (2011). Blocking early GABA depolarization with bumetanide results in permanent alterations in cortical circuits and sensorimotor gating deficits. *Cereb Cortex, 21*(3), 574-587. doi:10.1093/cercor/bhq124